GoodFood
Gluten-free recipes

10 9 8 7 6 5 4 3 2 1

Published in 2012 by BBC Books, an imprint of Ebury Publishing.
A Random House Group Company

Photographs © BBC Worldwide 2012
Recipes © BBC Worldwide 2012
Book design © Woodlands Books Ltd 2012
All recipes contained in this book first appeared in BBC Good Food magazine.

The Random House Group Limited
Reg. No. 954009

Addresses for companies within the Random House Group can be found at
www.randomhouse.co.uk

A CIP catalogue record for this book is available from the British Library.

The Random House Group Limited supports The Forest Stewardship Council (FSC®), the leading international
forest certification organisation. Our books carrying the FSC label are printed on FSC® certified paper.
FSC is the only forest certification scheme endorsed by the leading environmental organisations, including
Greenpeace. Our paper procurement policy can be found at www.randomhouse.co.uk/environment

To buy books by your favourite authors and register for offers visit www.randomhouse.co.uk

Colour reproduction by Dot Gradations Ltd, UK
Printed and bound by Firmengruppe APPL, aprinta druck, Wemding, Germany

Commissioning editor: Muna Reyal
Project editor: Sarah Watling
Designer: Kathryn Gammon
Production: Rebecca Jones
Picture researcher: Gabby Harrington

ISBN: 9781849905305

MIX
Paper from
responsible sources
FSC® C004592
www.fsc.org

Picture credits

BBC Good Food magazine would like to thank the following people for providing photos. While every effort has been made
to trace and acknowledge all photographers we should like to apologise should there be any errors or omissions.

Marie-Louise Avery p123; Peter Cassidy p83, p179, p181; Will Heap p41, p51, p75, p117, p125, p159; Gareth Morgans p19,
p119, p129, p147, p185; David Munns p21, p23, p27, p39, p69, p71, p77, p81, p103, p111, p133, p139, p165, p167, p171,
p195, p199; Myles New p11, p17, p25, p33, p35, p37, p53, p55, p59, p65, p73, p87, p91, p95, p97, p101, p105, p113, p121,
p141, p149, p153, p161, p163, p169, p175, p189, p191; Stuart Ovenden p49, p137; Lis Parsons p13, p15, p29, p43, p45, p47,
p57, p61, p63, p67, p131, p183, p193, p207; Maja Smend p31, p115, p127, p151, p155; Roger Stowell p143; Yuki Sugiura
p203; Debi Treloar p209; Simon Wallace p99; Philip Webb p85, p89, p93, p107, p109, p145, p157, p173, p177, p187, p197,
p201, p205, p211; Simon Wheeler p79

All the recipes in this book were created by the editorial team at Good Food and by regular contributors to BBC magazines.

everyday GoodFood
Gluten-free recipes

Editor **Sarah Cook**

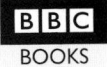

BOOKS

Contents

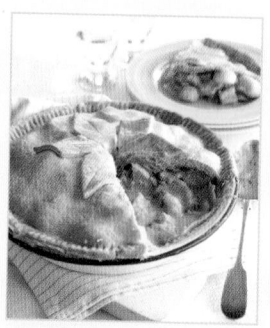 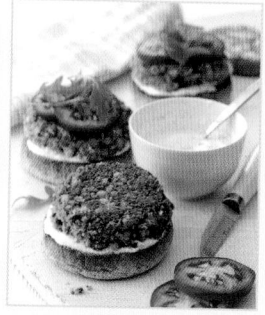 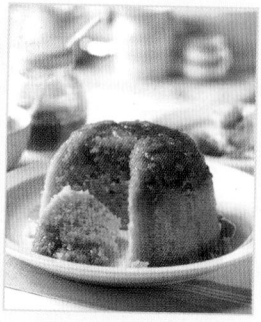

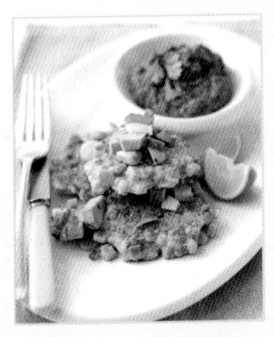

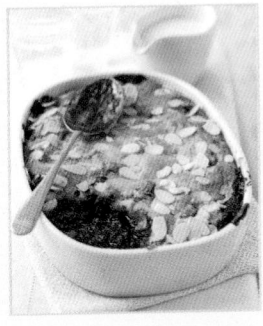

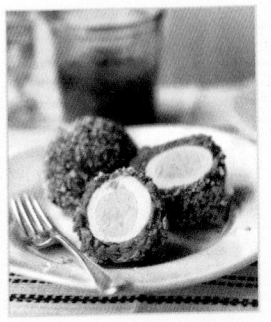

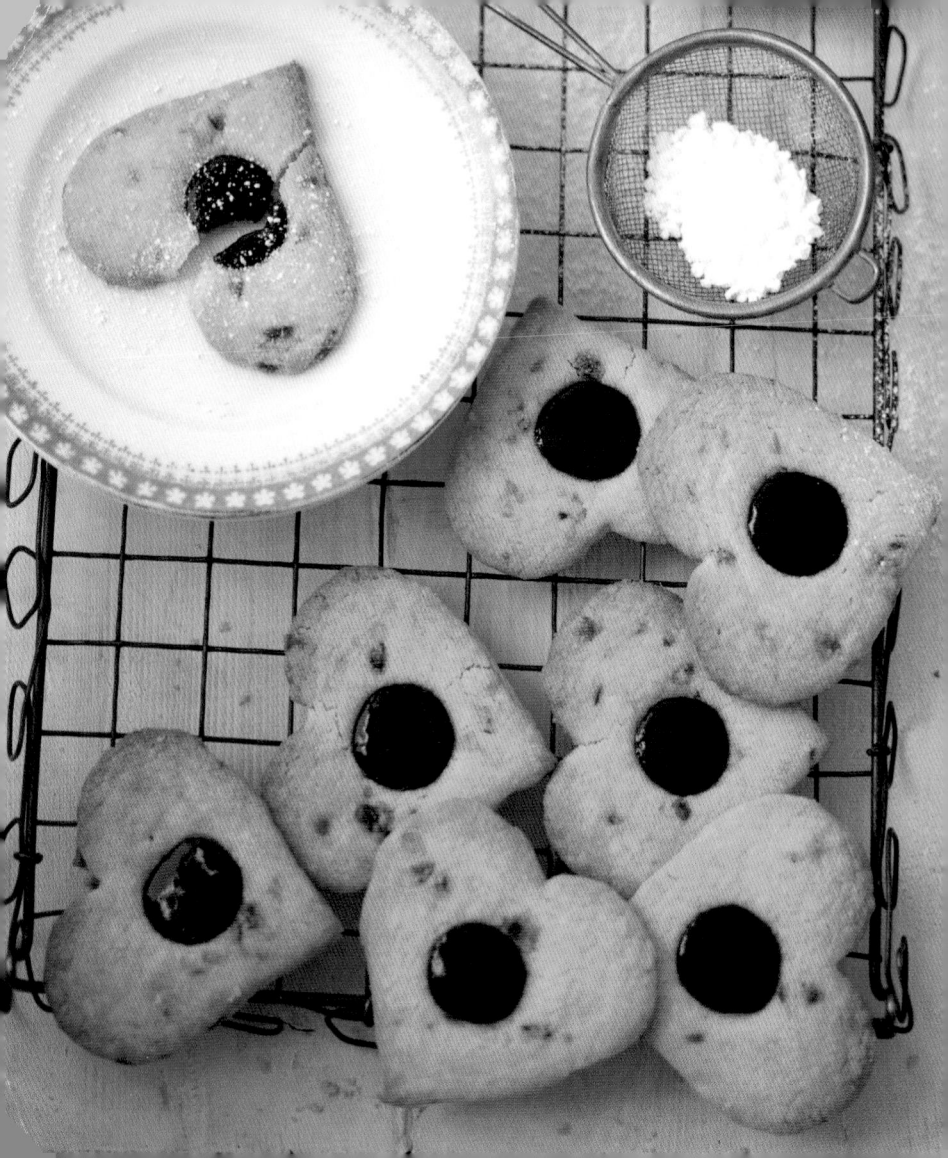

Introduction

No gluten? No problem, when you've got this handy little book in your kitchen. We've taken 101 of our best-loved recipes and made them gluten free so they can now be enjoyed by absolutely everyone.

Banned classics are back on the menu, so if you thought you'd never eat another yummy scone or Yorkshire pudding – think again! We've experimented with endless sauces, pastries and sponges to come up with lots of really good versions of all the foods you thought you'd said goodbye to forever.

There are heaps of simple supper and snack ideas to keep hungry kids happy, including homemade versions of favourites like fish fingers, burgers and pizza. Plus there's a chapter packed with ideas for more substantial options for those times when the whole family gets to sit down and eat together.

And because we know baking is one of the biggest challenges if you're gluten-free, we've devoted a big section to sweet and savoury cakes, bakes and bread – including a fantastic *Malted walnut seed loaf* on p194 that puts sandwiches back on the menu, and an amazing recipe for *Raspberry brownies* on p164 which we guarantee will fool anyone who tastes them into thinking they're the real deal!

As usual, every single recipe has been created and tested in the *Good Food* kitchen, so you can cook with confidence every time, knowing they'll be a big success. So what are you waiting for? Throw away that packet mix and open this clever book. Gluten-free cooking has never been so easy!

Sarah

Sarah

Notes and conversion tables

NOTES ON THE RECIPES

• Eggs are large in the UK and Australia and extra large in America unless stated otherwise.

• Wash fresh produce before preparation.

• Recipes contain nutritional analyses for 'sugar', which means the total sugar content including all natural sugars in the ingredients, unless otherwise stated.

OVEN TEMPERATURES

Gas	°C	°C Fan	°F	Oven temp.
¼	110	90	225	Very cool
½	120	100	250	Very cool
1	140	120	275	Cool or slow
2	150	130	300	Cool or slow
3	160	140	325	Warm
4	180	160	350	Moderate
5	190	170	375	Moderately hot
6	200	180	400	Fairly hot
7	220	200	425	Hot
8	230	210	450	Very hot
9	240	220	475	Very hot

APPROXIMATE WEIGHT CONVERSIONS

• All the recipes in this book list both imperial and metric measurements. Conversions are approximate and have been rounded up or down. Follow one set of measurements only; do not mix the two.

• Cup measurements, which are used by cooks in Australia and America, have not been listed here as they vary from ingredient to ingredient. Kitchen scales should be used to measure dry/solid ingredients.

Good Food is concerned about sustainable sourcing and animal welfare. Where possible humanely reared meats, sustainably caught fish (see fishonline. org for further information from the Marine Conservation Society) and free-range chickens and eggs are used when recipes are originally tested.

SPOON MEASURES

Spoon measurements are level unless otherwise specified.

- 1 teaspoon (tsp) = 5ml
- 1 tablespoon (tbsp) = 15ml
- 1 Australian tablespoon = 20ml (cooks in Australia should measure 3 teaspoons where 1 tablespoon is specified in a recipe)

APPROXIMATE LIQUID CONVERSIONS

metric	imperial	AUS	US
50ml	2fl oz	¼ cup	¼ cup
125ml	4fl oz	½ cup	½ cup
175ml	6fl oz	¾ cup	¾ cup
225ml	8fl oz	1 cup	1 cup
300ml	10fl oz/½ pint	½ pint	1¼ cups
450ml	16fl oz	2 cups	2 cups/1 pint
600ml	20fl oz/1 pint	1 pint	2½ cups
1 litre	35fl oz/1¾ pints	1¾ pints	1 quart

Peppered steak salad

This super-speedy salad is perfect for a Friday night in, when you want something tasty that doesn't keep you in the kitchen for ages.

TAKES 15 MINUTES • SERVES 4

2 tbsp olive oil
2 large, thin-cut sirloin steaks (about 175g/6oz each), trimmed of any fat
2 ripe avocados
4 tbsp mustard mayonnaise
2 handfuls gluten-free tortilla crisps
110g bag watercress, rocket & spinach salad

1 Rub a little of the oil over the steaks and generously season. Heat a griddle or frying pan until hot, then cook the steaks for 1–2 minutes each side, depending on the thickness of your steak and how you like it cooked. Remove from the pan and rest on a plate while you get the other ingredients ready.

2 Stone and peel the avocados, then thickly slice. Whisk the mustard mayo with the remaining oil, 4 teaspoons water and the resting juices from the steak to make a dressing.

3 Break the tortillas into pieces and slice the steak, trimming off any excess fat. Divide the salad between four plates, top with the avocado, tortilla pieces and sliced steak, and finally drizzle with dressing.

PER SERVING 453 kcals, protein 22g, carbs 16g, fat 34g, sat fat 6g, fibre 3g, sugar 2g, salt 0.64g

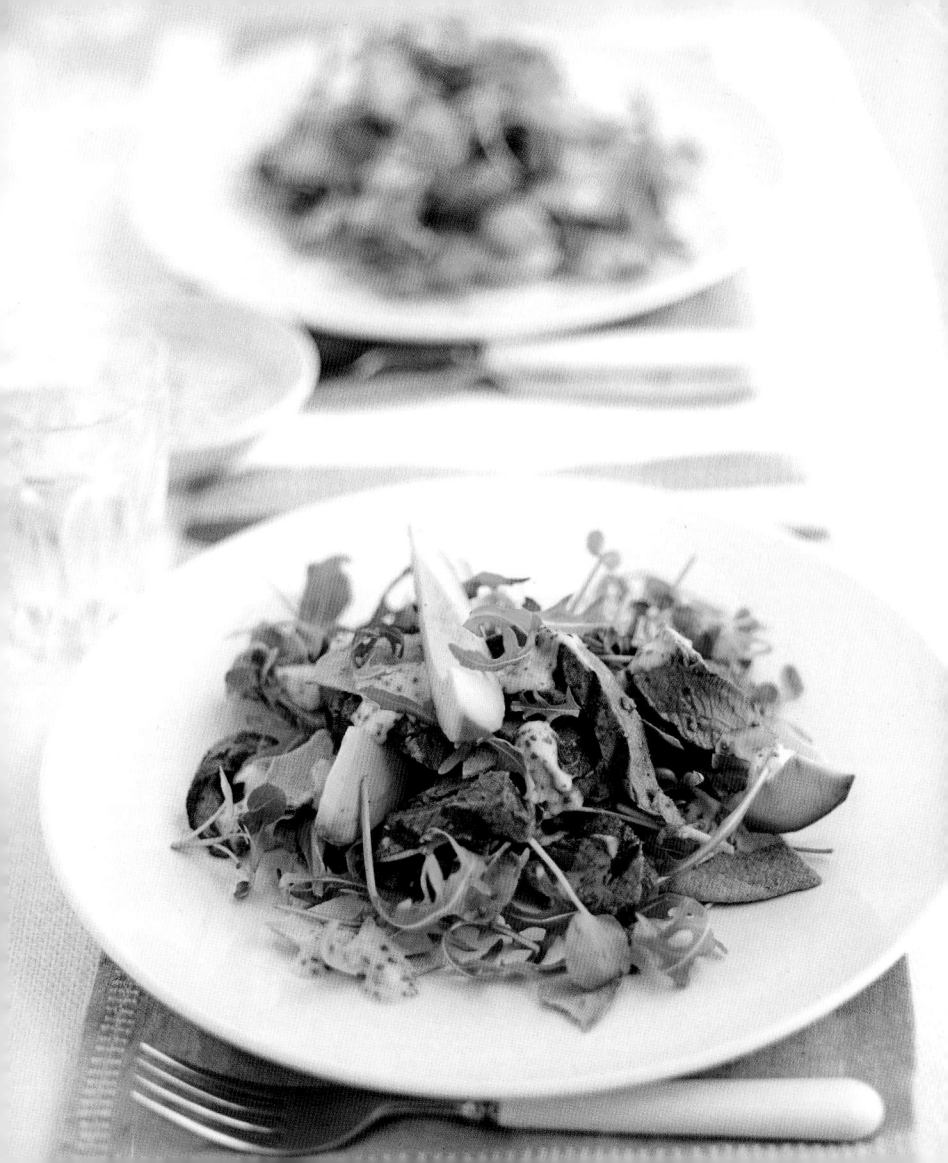

Sausage ball pasta bake

You may as well make double of this recipe to start with, as everybody is going to want second helpings!

TAKES 1 HOUR 5 MINUTES • SERVES 4

450g/1lb gluten-free sausages, meat squeezed from skins

50g/2oz gluten-free white bread, whizzed into crumbs

1 tbsp thyme or rosemary leaves, chopped

1 tbsp olive oil

500g carton passata

2 tbsp sun-dried tomato paste

300g/10oz gluten-free fusilli or other pasta shapes

½ small Savoy cabbage, cut into 1cm/½in-wide slices

250g ball mozzarella, cubed

2 tbsp freshly grated Parmesan

1 Put the sausagemeat, breadcrumbs and thyme or rosemary in a bowl and mix to combine. Shape into 20 small balls.

2 Heat the oil in a wide pan and cook the sausage balls for 10 minutes until nicely browned. Add the passata and tomato paste, cover and simmer gently for 20 minutes to make a sauce.

3 Meanwhile, cook the pasta according to the pack instructions, adding the cabbage for the final 5 minutes of cooking time. Drain the cabbage and pasta, toss with the sauce and spoon into a heatproof dish.

4 Heat oven to 200C/180C fan/gas 6. Push the mozzarella cubes into the top of the pasta. Sprinkle with Parmesan and bake for 15–20 minutes until bubbling and crusty.

PER SERVING 860 kcals, protein 41g, carbs 88g, fat 41g, sat fat 17g, fibre 7g, sugar 11g, salt 3.75g

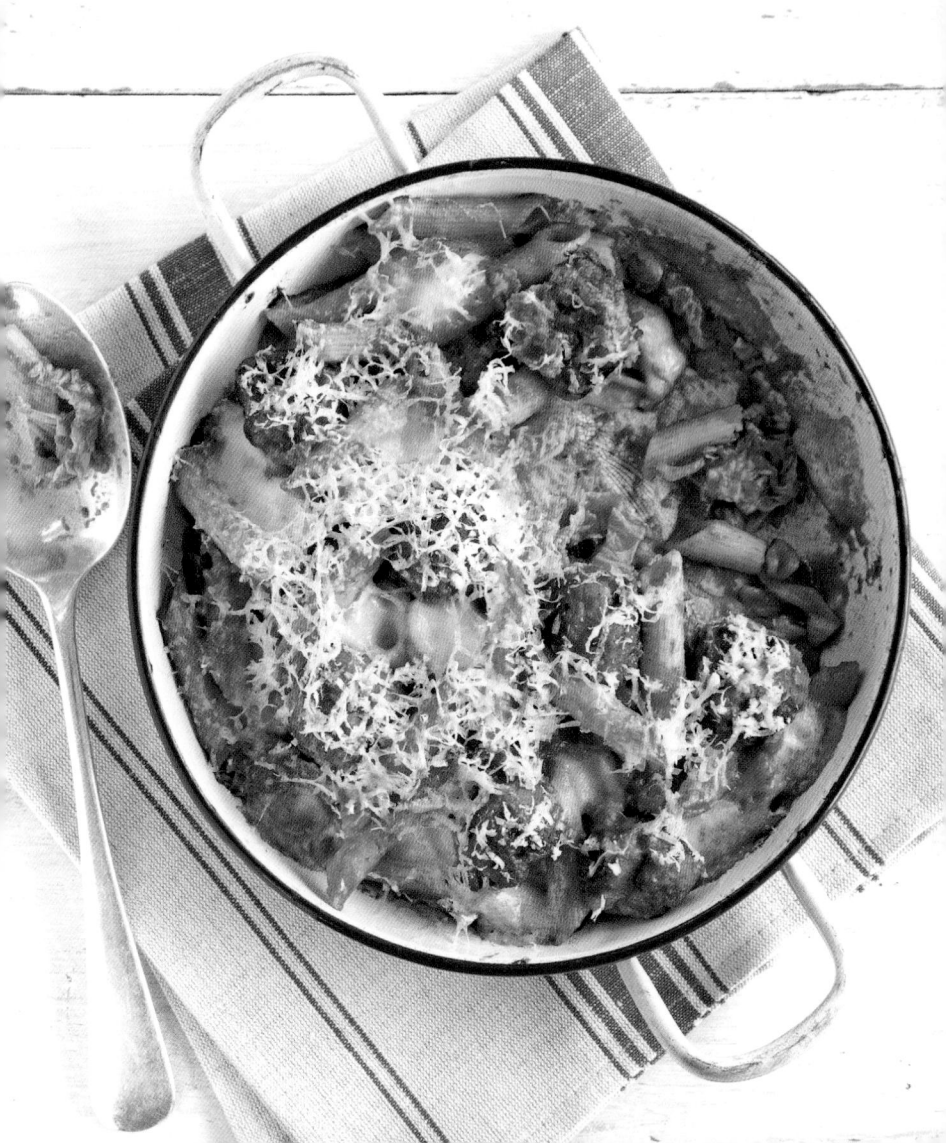

Mushroom rarebit with mash & thyme gravy

This is serious British comfort food for a chilly day, and meat eaters won't even notice it's vegetarian!

TAKES 1¾ HOURS • SERVES 4

1kg/2lb 4oz floury potatoes, chopped into chunks
50g/2oz butter
100ml/3½fl oz milk
4 large flat mushrooms, stems removed
olive oil, for brushing
1 medium onion, chopped
1 tbsp cornflour
75ml/2½fl oz gluten-free stout
140g/5oz mature Cheddar, grated
1 tsp gluten-free English mustard
2 eggs, beaten

FOR THE GRAVY

1 medium onion, chopped
2 tsp thyme leaves, plus extra to scatter
2 tbsp olive oil
1 tbsp cornflour
125ml/4fl oz white wine
300ml/½ pint gluten-free vegetable stock
2 tsp gluten-free yeast extract (we used Marmite)

1 Heat oven to 200C/180C fan/gas 6. Boil the potatoes until tender. Drain, return to the pan with half the butter and the milk. Mash; season and keep warm.

2 Meanwhile, brush the mushrooms with oil. Put gill-side up in a baking dish and bake for 15 minutes. Melt the remaining butter in a pan and fry the onion for 10–15 minutes. Add the flour for 1 minute. Reduce the heat, then add the stout, cheese, mustard and seasoning, stirring until the cheese has melted. Add the eggs and stir constantly until the mixture thickens but don't overcook. Spoon the rarebit mix into the mushroom caps.

3 For the gravy, fry the onion and thyme gently in the oil until the onion is soft. Add the cornflour and cook, stirring, for 2 minutes. Add the wine, stock and Marmite, then simmer until thick.

4 Just before serving, heat grill to high. Grill the mushrooms until the rarebit is puffed and golden. Scatter with thyme and serve with the mash and gravy.

PER SERVING 624 kcals, protein 23g, carbs 58g, fat 33g, sat fat 16g, fibre 6g, sugar 9g, salt 1.28g

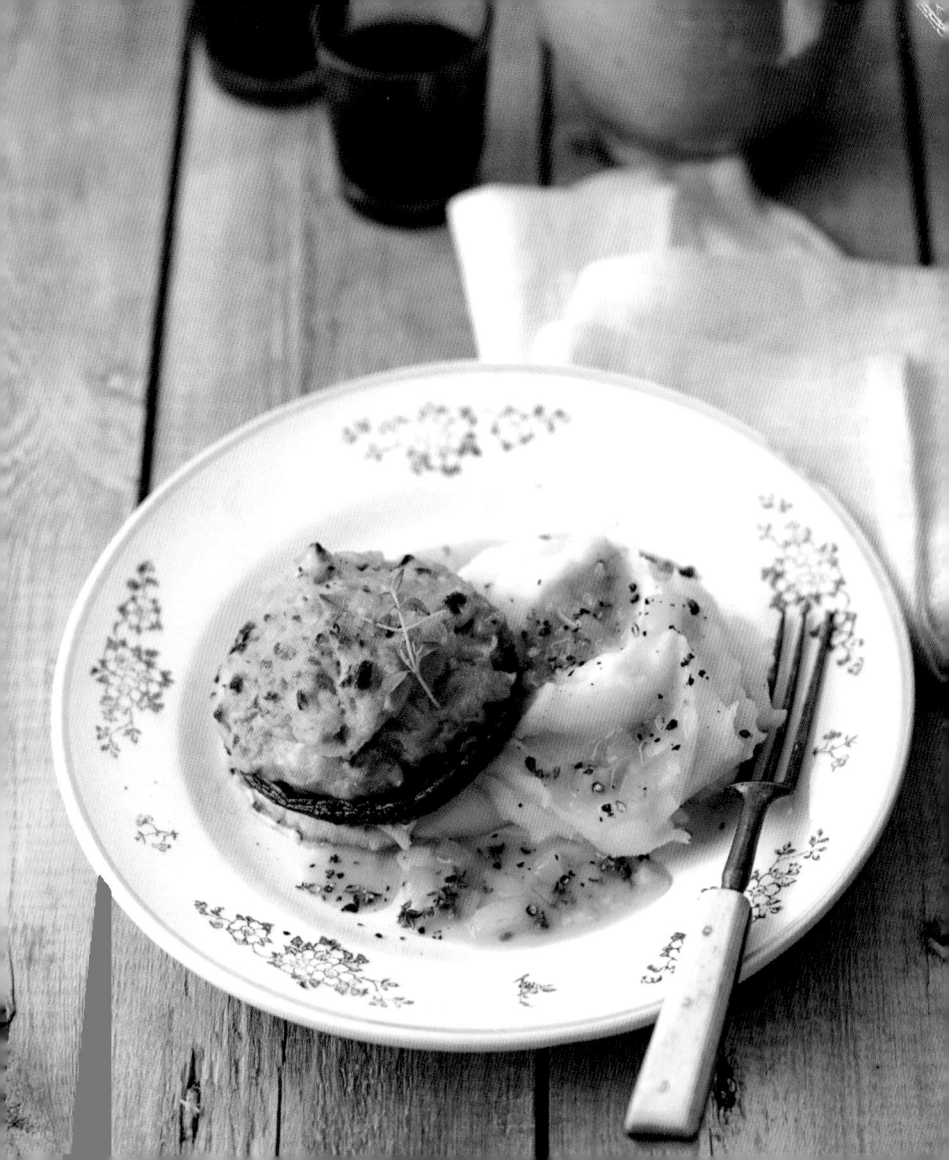

Spanish prawn & rice one pot

This easy one-pan can be on the dinner table in less than 30 minutes – just add a bag of salad.

TAKES 25 MINUTES • SERVES 4

1 onion, sliced

1 red and 1 green pepper, deseeded
and sliced

50g/2oz chorizo, sliced

2 garlic cloves, crushed

1 tbsp olive oil

250g/9oz easy cook basmati rice

400g can chopped tomatoes

500ml/18fl oz hot gluten-free vegetable
stock

200g/7oz raw peeled prawns,
defrosted if frozen

1 In a non-stick frying pan or shallow pan with a lid, fry the onion, peppers, chorizo and garlic in the oil over a high heat for 3 minutes. Stir in the rice and chopped tomatoes with the stock, cover, then cook over a high heat for 12–15 minutes.

2 Uncover, then stir – the rice should be almost tender. Stir in the prawns, with a splash more water if the rice is looking dry, then cook for another minute until the prawns are just pink and the rice is tender.

PER SERVING 356 kcals, protein 19g, carbs 59g, fat 7g, sat fat 2g, fibre 4g, sugar 7g, salt 0.85g

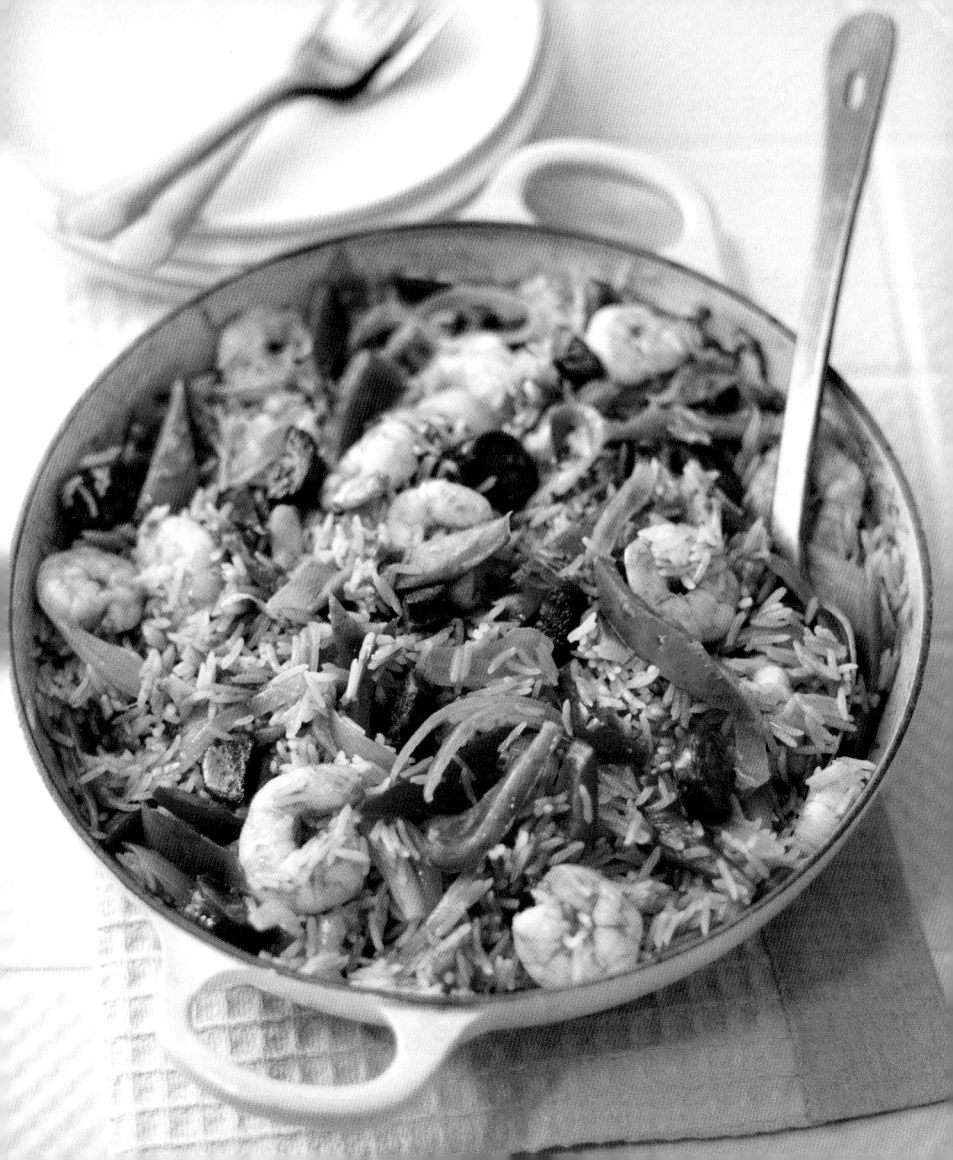

Cottage pie

To cook this pie from frozen, heat oven to 180C/160C fan/gas 4, cover with foil and cook for 2 hours. Then flash under the grill to brown.

TAKES 2 HOURS 20 MINUTES

● **SERVES 10**

3 tbsp olive oil

1.25kg/2lb 12oz minced beef

2 onions, finely chopped

3 carrots, chopped

3 celery sticks, chopped

2 garlic cloves, finely chopped

3 tbsp gluten-free plain flour

1 tbsp tomato purée

850ml/1½ pints gluten-free beef stock

4 tbsp Worcestershire sauce

few thyme sprigs

2 bay leaves

FOR THE MASH

1.8kg/4lb potatoes, chopped

225ml/8fl oz milk

25g/1oz butter

200g/7oz strong Cheddar, grated

1 Heat 1 tablespoon of the oil in a large saucepan and fry the mince in batches until browned. Add the remaining oil to the pan with the vegetables and soften. Add the garlic, flour and tomato purée, increase the heat and cook for a few minutes, then return the beef to the pan. Add the stock, Worcestershire sauce and herbs. Bring to a simmer and cook, uncovered, for 45 minutes. Season well, then discard the bay leaves and thyme stalks.

2 Meanwhile, make the mash. Boil the potatoes until tender. Drain well, then allow to steam-dry for a few minutes. Mash with the milk, butter, and three-quarters of the cheese, then season.

3 Spoon the meat into two ovenproof dishes. Spoon the mash over. Sprinkle on the remaining cheese. If eating straight away, heat oven to 220C/200C fan/gas 7 and cook for 25–30 minutes, or until the topping is golden. Or freeze for another time.

PER SERVING 600 kcals, protein 37g, carbs 40g, fat 34g, sat fat 16g, fibre 4g, sugar 7g, salt 1.15g

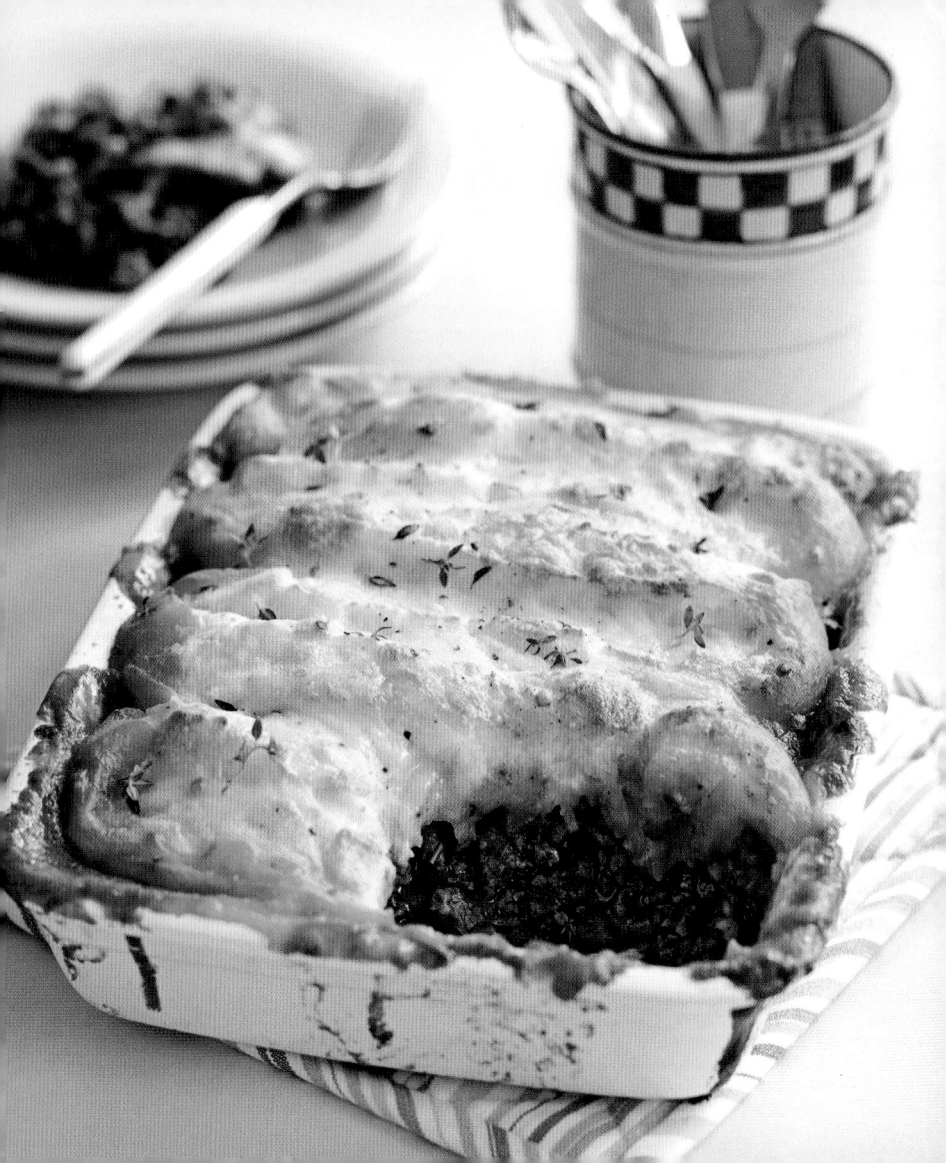

Black bean tostadas with avocado salsa

Gluten-free tortillas are available to buy online, but if you can't wait to make this then use gluten-free pitta bread instead – split in half to make it thinner and cook as below.

TAKES 25 MINUTES • SERVES 4

8 gluten-free corn tortillas or pitta breads, halved
2 tbsp olive oil
1 onion, chopped
3 garlic cloves, chopped
1 tbsp each smoked paprika and ground cumin
5 tbsp cider vinegar
3 tbsp clear honey
3 × 400g cans black beans, rinsed and drained
choose a few toppings such as chopped tomatoes, sliced red onion, diced avocado, sliced jalapeño peppers, coriander sprigs
crème fraîche or Tabasco chipotle sauce, to serve

1 Heat oven to 200C/180C fan/gas 6. Brush the tortillas or pittas with a little of the oil and put in a single layer on baking sheets. Cook for 8 minutes until crisp.

2 In a large frying pan, heat the remaining oil. Add the onion and garlic, and cook for 5 minutes. Add the spices, vinegar and honey. Cook for 2 minutes more. Add the beans and some seasoning, and heat through.

3 Remove from the heat and mash the beans gently with the back of your spoon to a chunky purée. Spread some beans over the crispy corn tortillas or pittas, scatter with your choice of toppings and add a spoonful of crème fraîche to cool down, or a splash of chipotle Tabasco to spice it up.

PER SERVING 675 kcals, protein 27g, carbs 91g, fat 17g, sat fat 7g, fibre 15g, sugar 18g, salt 0.6g

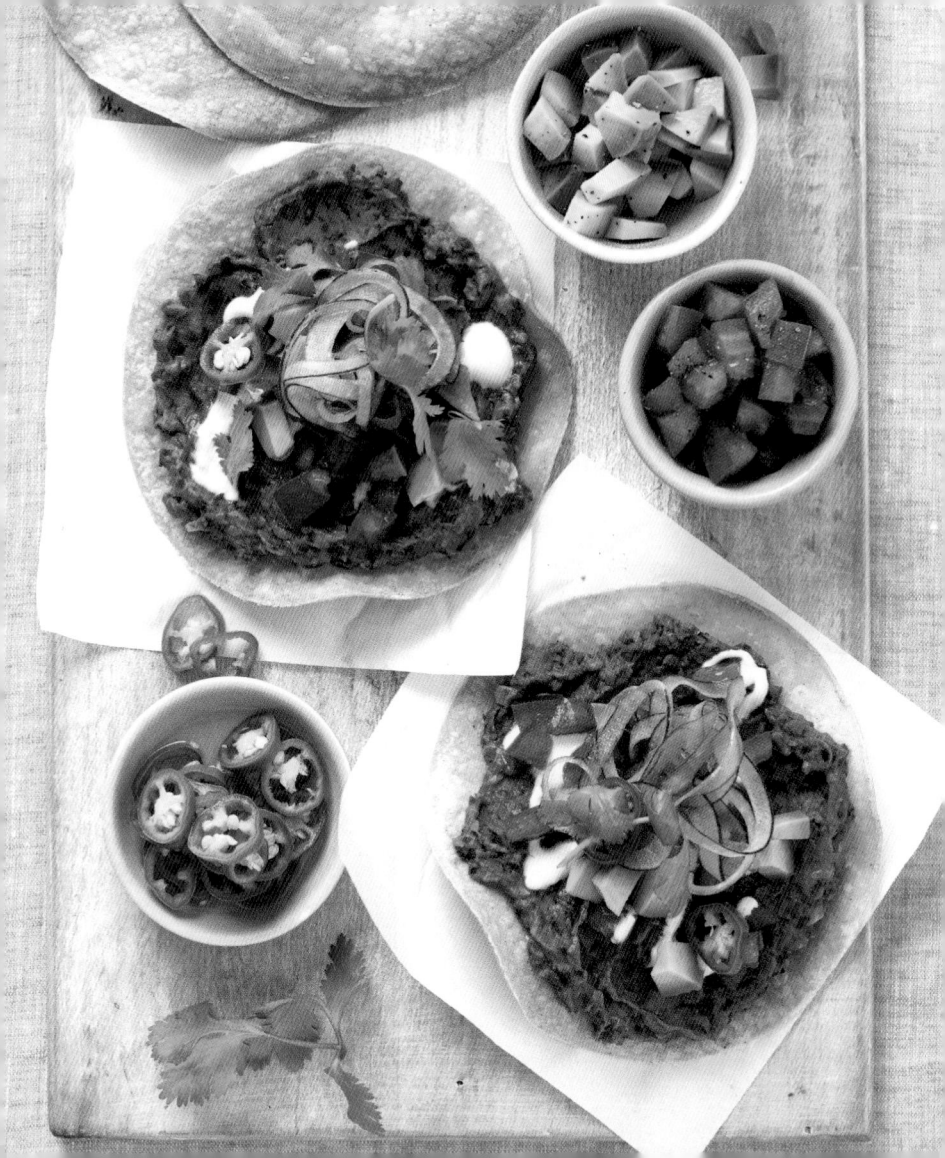

Warm quinoa salad with grilled halloumi

Quinoa is brilliant for gluten-free vegetarians as it contains good levels of protein, and is also an excellent source of calcium, iron and B vitamins.

TAKES 40 MINUTES • SERVES 3

3 tbsp extra virgin olive oil

1 small red onion, sliced

1 large roasted pepper from a jar, thickly sliced, or handful ready-roasted sliced peppers

200g/7oz quinoa

500ml/18fl oz gluten-free vegetable stock

small bunch flat-leaf parsley, roughly chopped

zest and juice 1 lemon

large pinch sugar

250g pack halloumi, cut into 6 slices

1 Heat 1 tablespoon of the oil in a medium pan. Cook the onion and pepper for a few minutes, then add the quinoa and cook for a further 3 minutes. Add the stock, cover and turn the heat down to a simmer. Cook for 15 minutes or until soft, then stir half the parsley through the salad and set aside. Heat the grill.

2 Mix the lemon zest and juice with the remaining parsley and oil, and the sugar and a large pinch of salt to make a dressing.

3 Grill the halloumi until both sides are golden and crisp. Serve the salad with the grilled halloumi and the dressing poured over everything.

PER SERVING 603 kcals, protein 28g, carbs 40g, fat 37g, sat fat 16g, fibre 1g, sugar 7g, salt 3.1g

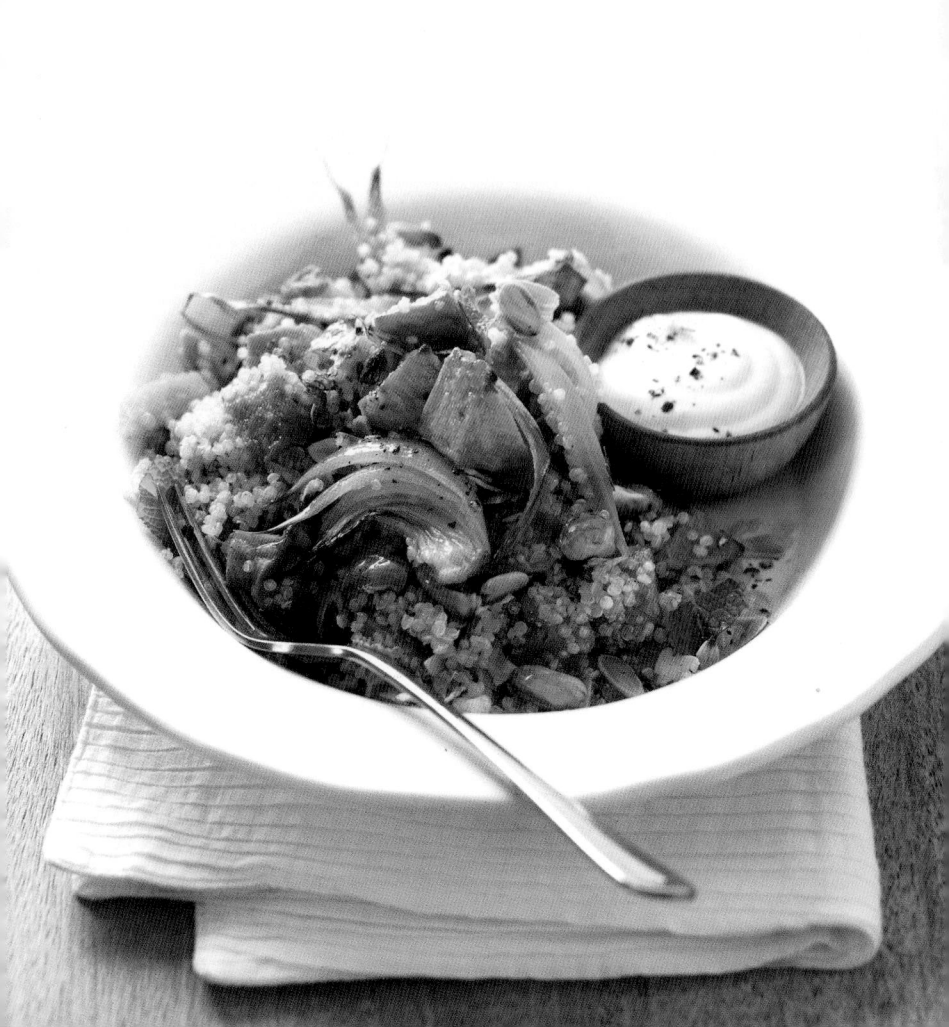

Crisp-crumb fishcakes

These low-fat fishcakes will freeze beautifully for up to 2 months. Defrost in the fridge for 24 hours then cook as below.

TAKES 1 HOUR 5 MINUTES

● **MAKES 8**

700g/1lb 9oz floury potatoes, cut into large chunks
600ml/1 pint milk
800g/1lb 12oz boneless white fish, skin on
1 tbsp wholegrain mustard
5 tbsp mayonnaise or tartare sauce
6 spring onions, finely sliced
zest 1 lemon
handful parsley, roughly chopped

FOR THE COATING

100g/4oz gluten-free plain flour, well seasoned, plus extra for dusting
1 egg, beaten
175g/6oz gluten-free white bread, whizzed into crumbs
2 tbsp sunflower oil, for frying

1 Boil the potatoes in a pan until tender. Put the milk in a frying pan; season. Bring just to boiling, then add the fish, skin-side down. Gently cook for 5–10 minutes.

2 Remove the fish from the milk, discard the skin and milk, then wipe out the pan. Break the fish into large flakes, then drain on kitchen paper. When the potatoes are done, drain, return them to the pan, then briefly heat on the hob to steam-dry. Mash well, stir in the mustard, mayo or tartare sauce, spring onions, lemon zest, parsley and flaked fish, then season well.

3 Using floured hands, divide the mixture into eight, then shape each portion into a patty. Put the flour, beaten egg and breadcrumbs on three large plates. Dip each fishcake into the flour, then the egg and finally the breadcrumbs, shaking off any excess as you go.

4 Heat the oil in the frying pan, then fry the fishcakes for about 3 minutes on each side. Keep the first batch warm in the oven while you finish cooking the rest.

PER FISHCAKE 371 kcals, protein 25g, carbs 42g, fat 12g, sat fat 2g, fibre 2g, sugar 2g, salt 0.8g

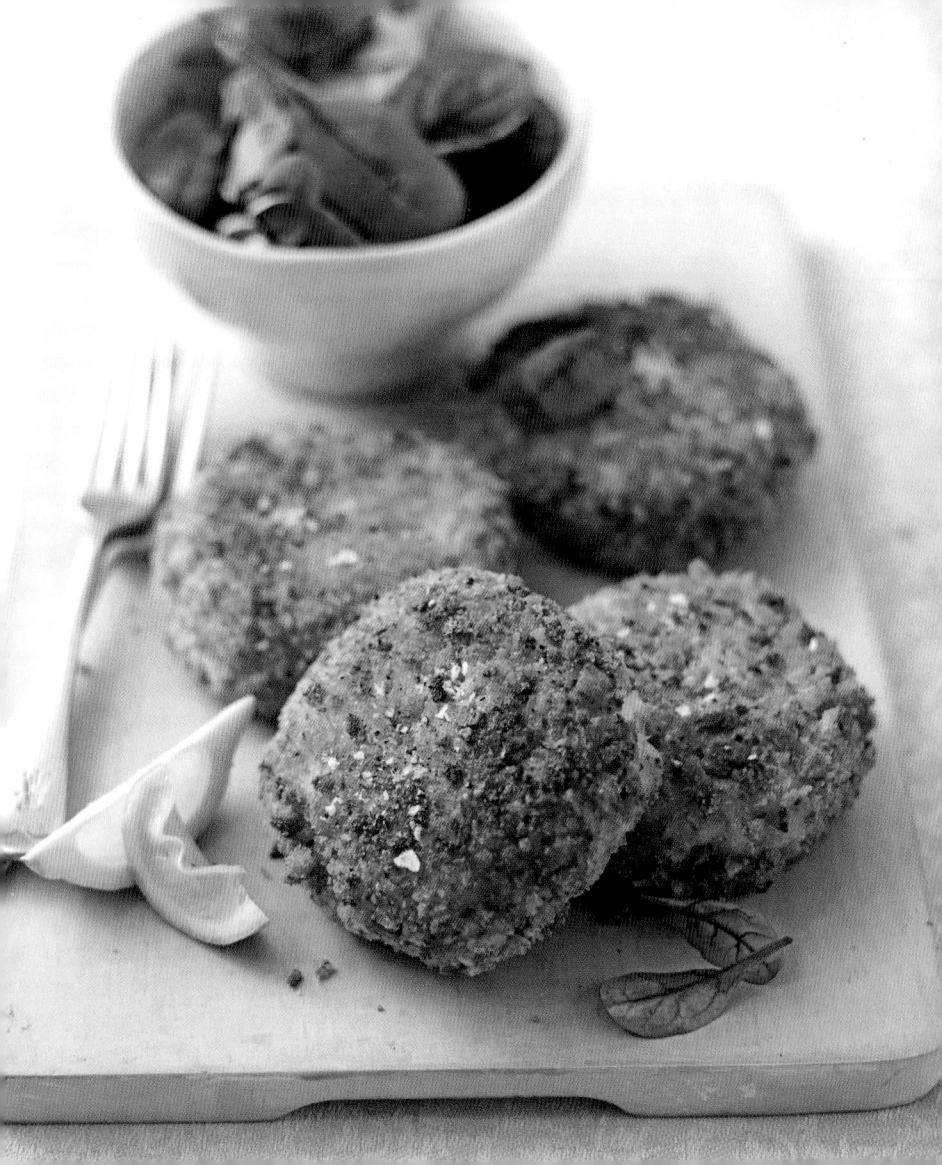

Macaroni cheese

Not only is this macaroni cheese gluten-free, it's also better for you than a traditional recipe. The chilli doesn't really spice it up too much, just adds an extra burst of flavour.

TAKES 1 HOUR 5 MINUTES ● SERVES 4

550ml/19fl oz semi-skimmed milk
25g/1oz cornflour
1 heaped tsp English mustard powder
1 large garlic clove, finely chopped
generous pinch crushed dried chillies
140g/5oz extra mature Cheddar, grated
25g/1oz gluten-free bread, whizzed
  into crumbs
200g/7oz gluten-free macaroni
1 bunch spring onions, finely sliced
25g/1oz Parmesan, grated
150ml/¼ pint buttermilk
450g/1lb mixed tomatoes, cherry
  tomatoes halved, large ones sliced

1 Mix 3 tablespoons of the milk with the cornflour and mustard, and set aside. Heat the remaining milk with the garlic until it is just coming to the boil. Remove from the heat and add the chillies.

2 Mix a handful of the Cheddar with the breadcrumbs. Heat oven to 200C/180C fan/gas 6.

3 Cook macaroni according to pack instructions, adding spring onions for the final 2 minutes.

4 Stir the cornflour mix into the warm infused milk. Return the pan to the heat, bring to the boil, stirring, until thickened and smooth. Remove from the heat and stir in Parmesan, most of the remaining Cheddar, buttermilk and seasoning.

5 Drain the macaroni then stir into the sauce. Pour into an ovenproof dish. Lay the tomatoes over the top then scatter over the cheesy breadcrumbs and the rest of the cheese. Bake for about 25 minutes.

PER SERVING 503 kcals, protein 26g, carbs 62g, fat 19g, sat fat 11g, fibre 3g, sugar 14g, salt 1.15g

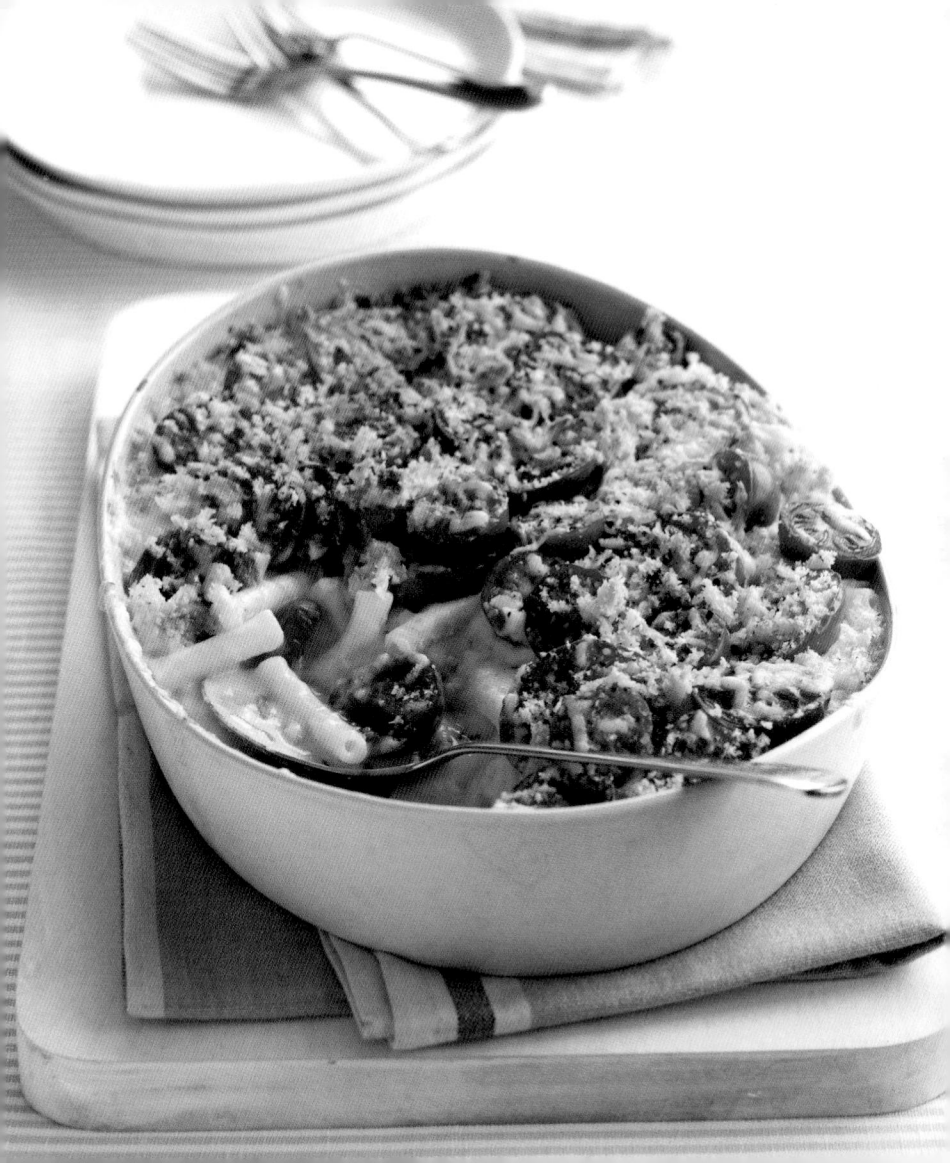

Chicken, ham, leek & roast potato pie

A brilliant way to use up leftover roast potatoes. If you don't have any, they're readily available from the chiller cabinet in supermarkets.

TAKES 1 HOUR 40 MINUTES

● **SERVES 4, WITH LEFTOVERS**

2 tbsp olive oil

400g/14oz skinless chicken breasts, cut into small chunks

140g/5oz thick-sliced ham, roughly chopped

leftover roast potatoes (about 450g/1lb), cut into large chunks

2 leeks, trimmed and sliced

1 tbsp cornflour

200ml/7fl oz white wine

400ml/14fl oz gluten-free chicken stock

2 tbsp crème fraîche

FOR THE PASTRY

250g/9oz gluten-free flour, plus extra for dusting

1 tsp xanthan gum

120g/4½oz butter, diced

2 eggs, beaten separately

1 For the pastry, put the flour, gum, butter and ½ teaspoon salt into a food processor and whizz until there are no lumps left. Dribble one of the eggs into the food processor while whizzing, until the pastry starts to come together. Add 1 tablespoon water at a time if it is too dry. Knead the dough for a few minutes, then wrap in cling film and chill for 30 minutes.

2 Heat half the oil in a frying pan and brown the chicken. Tip into a pie dish, then scatter over the ham and potatoes.

3 Heat the remaining oil and soften the leeks, then stir in the cornflour. Stir in the wine and stock and boil rapidly to a thick sauce. Stir in the crème fraîche and seasoning. Pour over the pie filling.

4 Roll out pastry on a lightly floured surface and place on top of the pie. Trim and crimp the edges with a fork. Decorate with trimmings, if you like, and brush with the second egg.

5 Heat oven to 200C/180C fan/gas 6 and cook for 30–40 minutes, until hot through.

PER SERVING 956 kcals, protein 46g, carbs 82g, fat 50g, sat fat 19g, fibre 5g, sugar 6g, salt 2.31g

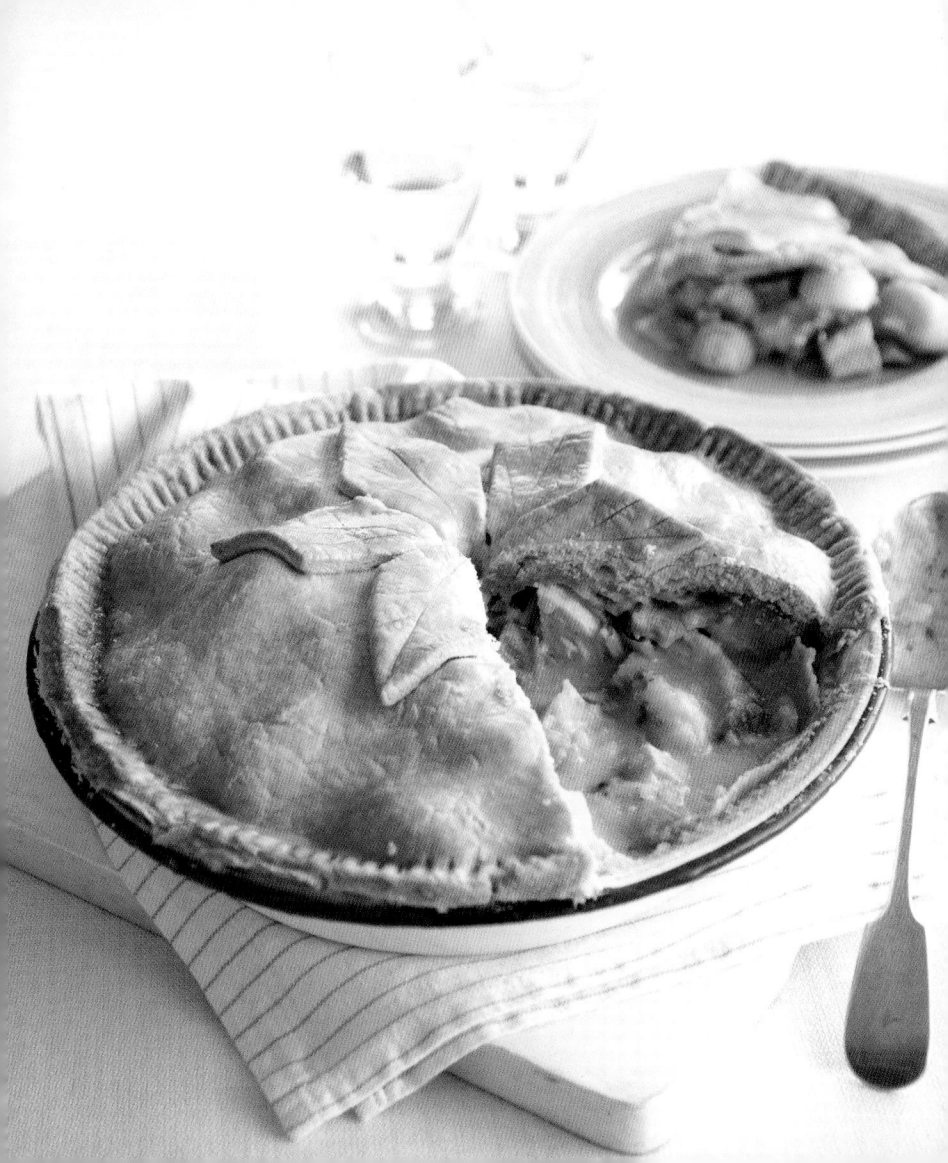

Garden herb pesto

Ready-made sauces often can't guarantee to be gluten-free because of the manufacturing process.

TAKES 10 MINUTES ● SERVES 6–8

100g/4oz mixed soft herbs – choose a mixture of basil, flat-leaf or English parsley, mint, chives, dill, whatever you have in your garden or fridge, plus extra to garnish (optional)

300ml/½ pint full-fat crème fraîche

100g/4oz Parmesan, grated, plus extra to garnish

100g/4oz pine nuts, toasted, plus extra to garnish

50g/2oz gluten-free spaghetti or linguine or 100g/4oz other gluten-free pasta shapes per person

1 Put the herbs, crème fraîche and Parmesan in a food processor and whizz together. Add the pine nuts and pulse so they are just a little chopped. Season really, really well, then divide any you want to freeze among ice-cube trays using a couple of teaspoons. Wrap in cling film and freeze.

2 To serve, cook the pasta according to the pack instructions. Drain, then stir in the fresh pesto. If you are using frozen cubes, pop one or two pesto ice cubes per person into the pasta pan. Tip the drained pasta back on top, put the lid on and leave for 10 minutes. Stir the melted pesto into the pasta, then serve topped with more Parmesan, a few pine nuts and extra herbs, if you like.

PER SERVING (6) 381 kcals, protein 10g, carbs 3g, fat 37g, sat fat 17g, fibre 1g, sugar 2g, salt none

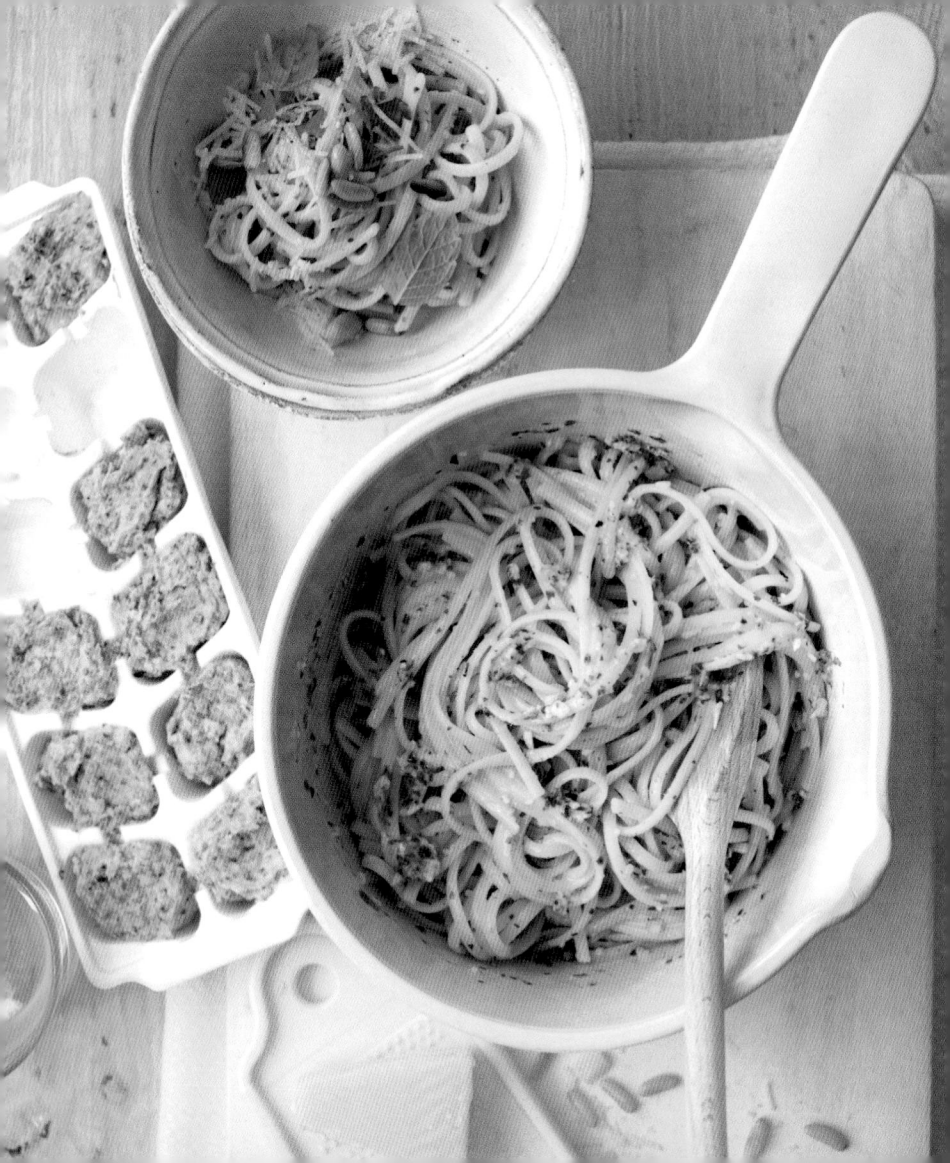

Beef stew with horseradish dumplings

This is easy, delicious and dead simple. Just put it all together, then into the oven it goes. Use a cut like shin or neck with real flavour, and let it cook slow and long.

TAKES 3½ HOURS ● SERVES 8

2kg/4lb 8oz beef shin, neck or stewing
    steak, chopped into large chunks
25g/1oz vegetable oil
500g/1lb 2oz shallots
2 gluten-free beef stock cubes,
    crumbled
1 tbsp Worcestershire sauce
1 potato (about 200g/7oz), peeled and
    grated
1–2 tbsp cornflour

FOR THE DUMPLINGS

70g/2½oz each butter and lard, frozen
350g/12oz gluten-free self-raising flour
    (check it contains xanthan gum,
    if not add 3 tsp xanthan gum)
2 tbsp creamed horseradish

1 Heat oven to 140C/120C fan/gas 1. Brown the beef in the oil, in a casserole with a lid. Spoon the beef into another dish as it is browned. Add the shallots and cook for 10 minutes. Return the meat with any juices, the stock cubes, Worcestershire sauce, grated potato and 1 litre/1¾ pints boiling water. Scraping the bottom of the pan to extract all the flavour, bring to the boil. Cover, transfer to the oven and cook for 2½ hours.

2 Just before the beef cooking time is up, make the dumplings. Grate the lard and butter into a bowl with the flour. Whisk the horseradish into 175ml/6fl oz cold water, then stir into the flour mix to form a heavy dough. Roll the dough into balls.

3 Make a paste with the cornflour and a little of the stew sauce. Whisk back into the stew, and sit on the hob to thicken. Pop the dumplings into the casserole dish, leave off the lid and return to the oven. Increase heat to 200C/180C fan/gas 6 and cook for 25–30 minutes.

PER SERVING 752 kcals, protein 64g, carbs 48g, fat 35g, sat fat 15g, fibre 3g, sugar 3g, salt 1.16g

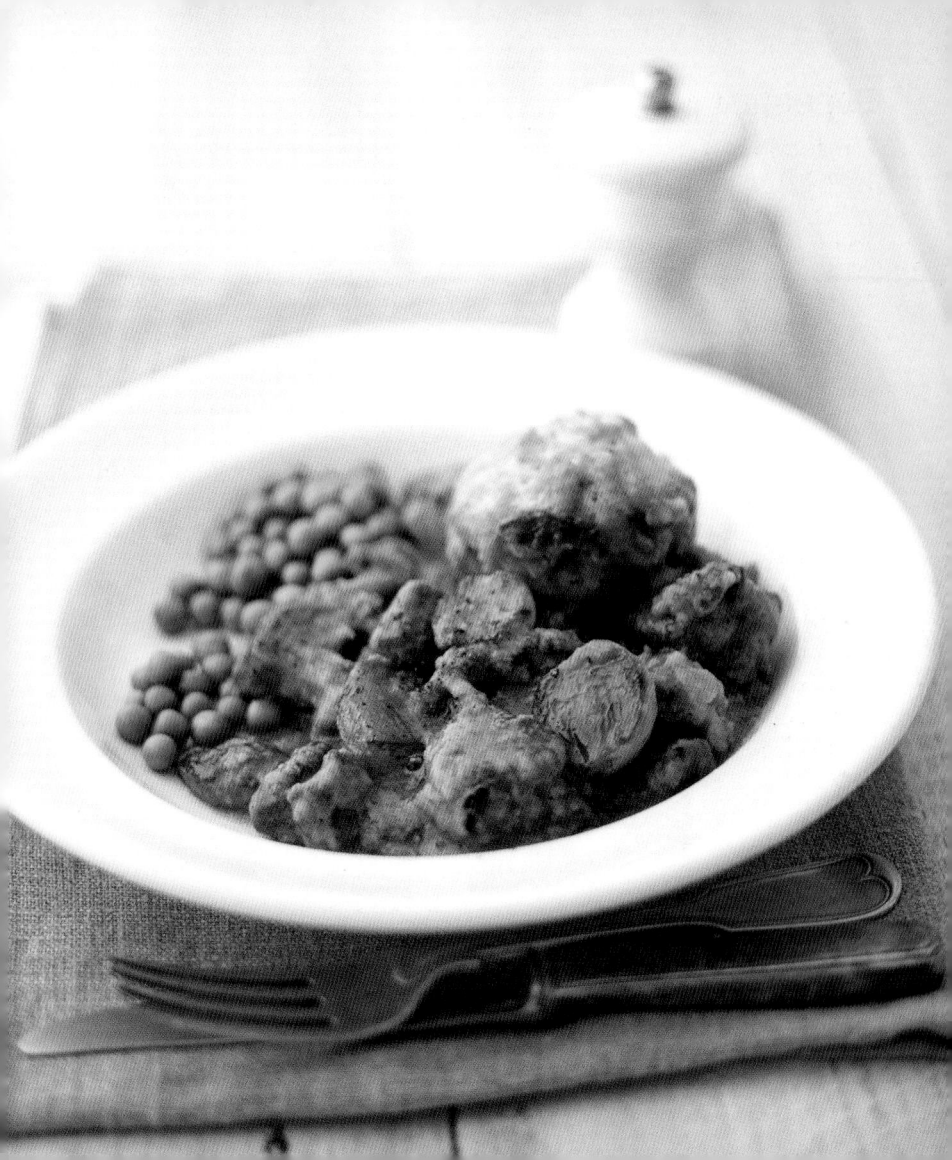

Super-fast pad Thai

Try to get the wide ribbon-like rice noodles as they're more authentic than the thin noodles in a pad Thai.

TAKES 15 MINUTES • SERVES 4

200g/7oz rice noodles
140g/5oz frozen peas
200g/7oz frozen prawns
2 tbsp sunflower oil
100g/4oz beansprouts
small bunch spring onions, sliced
2 eggs, beaten
3 tbsp roasted peanuts, chopped
2 tbsp gluten-free soy sauce or tamari
2 tbsp sweet chilli sauce
small bunch coriander, leaves only,
   to garnish

1 Bring a pan of water to the boil, add the noodles and cook for 3 minutes, adding the peas and prawns for the final minute. Drain well.

2 Heat the oil in a large frying pan. Fry the noodles, prawns, peas, beansprouts and spring onions, tossing to coat in the oil, for a few minutes. Push everything to one side of the pan and pour in the eggs. Stir until cooked, then mix everything well.

3 Toss through the peanuts, soy or tamari and sweet chilli sauce so everything is combined. Scatter with the coriander and serve.

PER SERVING 405 kcals, protein 23g, carbs 51g, fat 14g, sat fat 3g, fibre 4g, sugar 7g, salt 2.7g

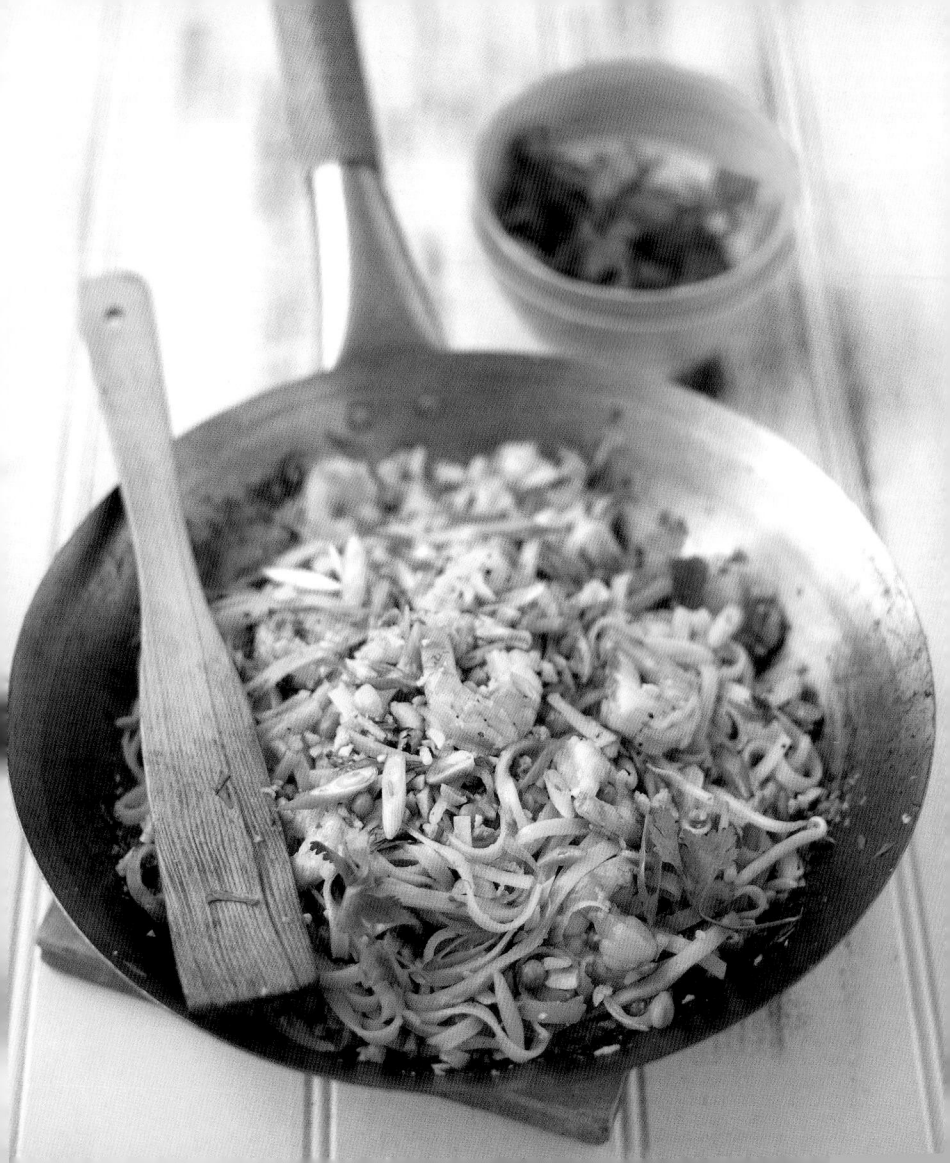

Fish pies

If you're making the pies ahead, cool quickly then cover and chill or freeze – but you'll need to bake them for a little bit longer to heat them through thoroughly from cold.

TAKES 1½ HOURS • SERVES 4

200g/7oz smoked haddock
200g/7oz sustainable white firm fish fillets
200g/7oz salmon fillets
600ml/1 pint semi-skimmed milk
25g/1oz cornflour
1 heaped tsp English mustard powder
500g/1lb 2oz Maris Piper potatoes, chopped
25g/1oz butter
good grating whole nutmeg
100g/4oz peeled cooked king prawns
140g/5oz frozen peas
4 hard-boiled eggs, quartered
small handful each parsley and dill
juice ½ lemon

1 Put all the fish in a wide pan. Pour over 500ml/18fl oz of the milk, cover and bring to a simmer. Cook gently for 5–8 minutes. Keep checking and remove from the heat as soon as the fish is cooked through and flaking. Lift out the fish and set aside.

2 Put the cornflour and mustard powder in a bowl and mix to a paste with a little of the poaching milk. Whisk back into the milk, then bring to the boil, stirring constantly, until thickened and smooth.

3 Put the potatoes in a pan and cover with cold water. Bring to the boil, then simmer for 10–15 minutes. Drain, tip back into the pan and mash with the butter, remaining milk and a grating of nutmeg.

4 Heat oven to 200C/180C fan/gas 6. Remove the skin from the fish and flake it into big chunks then stir into the sauce with the prawns, peas, eggs, parsley, dill and lemon juice. Season, then divide among four individual pie dishes.

5 Pipe or spoon the mash on top. Bake for 20–30 minutes.

PER SERVING 620 kcals, protein 49g, carbs 36g, fat 31g, sat fat 14g, fibre 4.8g, sugar 9g, salt 1.9g

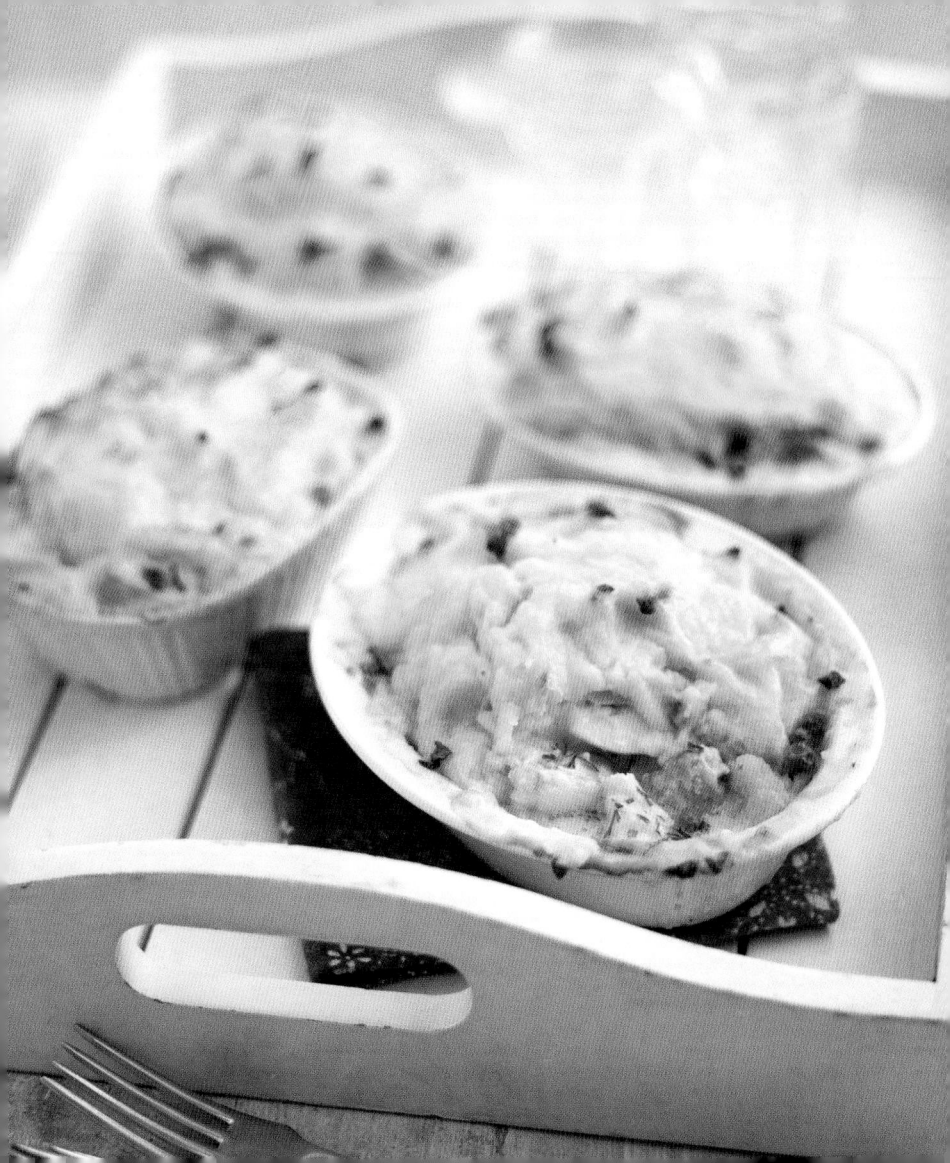

Summer vegetable curry

Lentils are a great gluten-free way of bulking up curries and stews – keep a pack, plus a jar of gluten-free Thai curry paste, in your storecupboard at all times.

TAKES 45 MINUTES • SERVES 4

1–2 tbsp gluten-free Thai red curry paste (depending on taste)
500ml/18fl oz gluten-free vegetable stock
2 onions, chopped
1 aubergine, diced
75g/2½oz red split lentils
200ml can reduced-fat coconut milk
2 red or yellow peppers, deseeded and cut into chunks
140g/5oz frozen peas
100g bag baby leaf spinach, roughly chopped
brown basmati rice and mango chutney, to serve

1 Heat the curry paste in a large non-stick pan with a splash of the stock. Add the onions and fry for 5 minutes until starting to soften. Stir in the aubergine and cook for a further 5 minutes – add a little more stock if it starts to stick.

2 Add the lentils, coconut milk and the rest of the stock, and simmer for 15 minutes or until the lentils are tender. Add the peppers and cook for 5–10 minutes more. Stir through the peas and spinach, and cook until the spinach has just wilted. Serve the curry with rice and mango chutney.

PER SERVING 207 kcals, protein 10g, carbs 28g, fat 7g, sat fat 4g, fibre 7g, sugar 12g, salt 0.49g

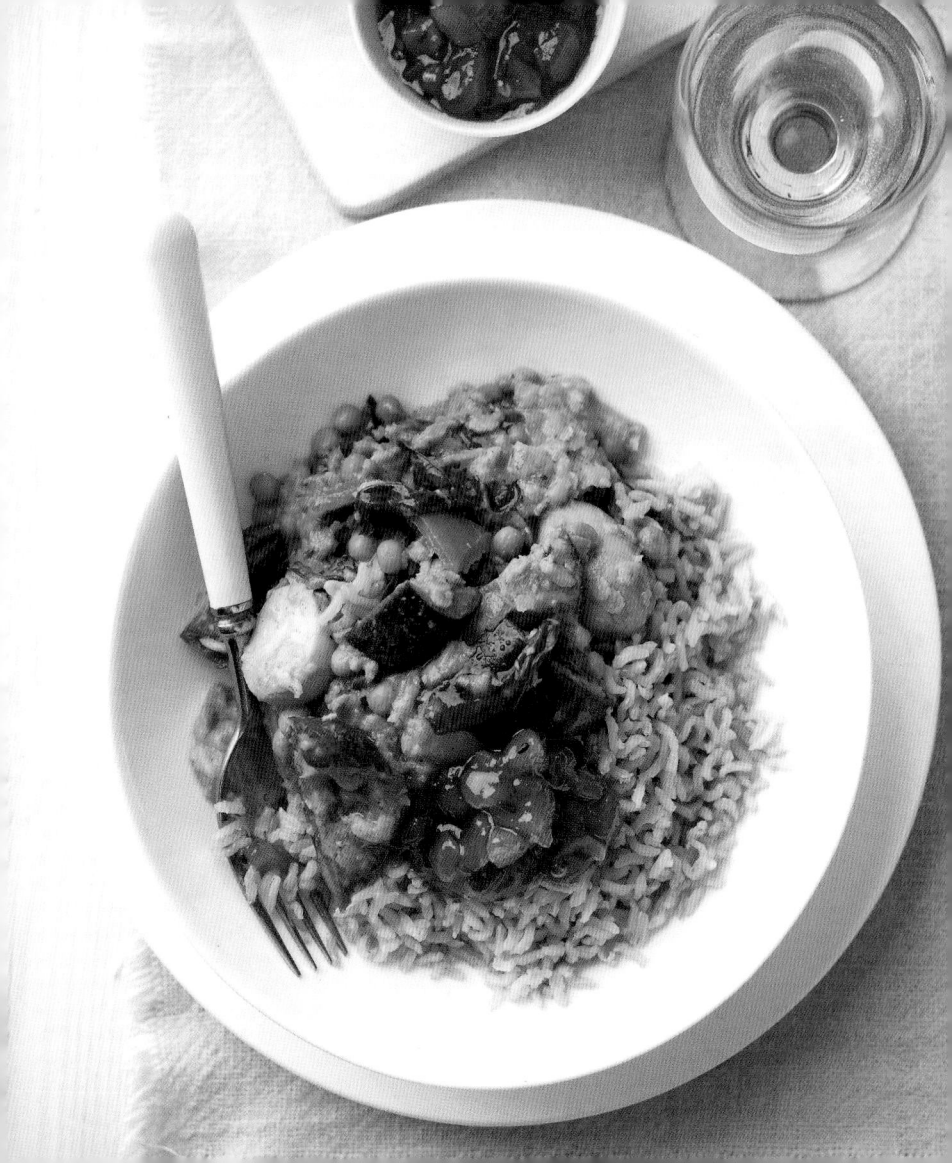

Cheeseburgers

This makes a lot of burgers, but if you're going to the effort of making your own it's worth getting a whole batch done and sticking half in the freezer for another time.

TAKES 40 MINUTES ● MAKES 12

1kg/2lb 4oz minced beef

300g/10oz gluten-free bread, whizzed into crumbs

140g/5oz extra-mature or mature Cheddar, grated

4 tbsp Worcestershire sauce

1 small bunch parsley, finely chopped

2 eggs, beaten

TO SERVE

split gluten-free burger buns, sliced tomatoes, red onion slices, lettuce, tomato sauce, coleslaw, wedges or fries

1 Crumble the mince into a large bowl, then tip in the breadcrumbs, cheese, Worcestershire sauce, parsley and eggs with 1 teaspoon ground pepper and 1–2 teaspoons salt. Mix with your hands to combine everything thoroughly.

2 Shape the mix into 12 burgers. Chill until ready to cook, for up to 24 hours, or freeze for up to 3 months. Just stack between squares of baking parchment to stop the burgers sticking together, then wrap well. Defrost overnight in the fridge before cooking.

3 To cook the burgers, heat the grill. Grill burgers for 6–8 minutes on each side until cooked through. Meanwhile, warm as many buns as you need on a foil-covered baking sheet below the grilling burgers. Let everyone assemble their own, served with their favourite accompaniments.

PER BURGER 343 kcals, protein 24g, carbs 20g, fat 19g, sat fat 9g, fibre 1g, sugar 1g, salt 1.05g

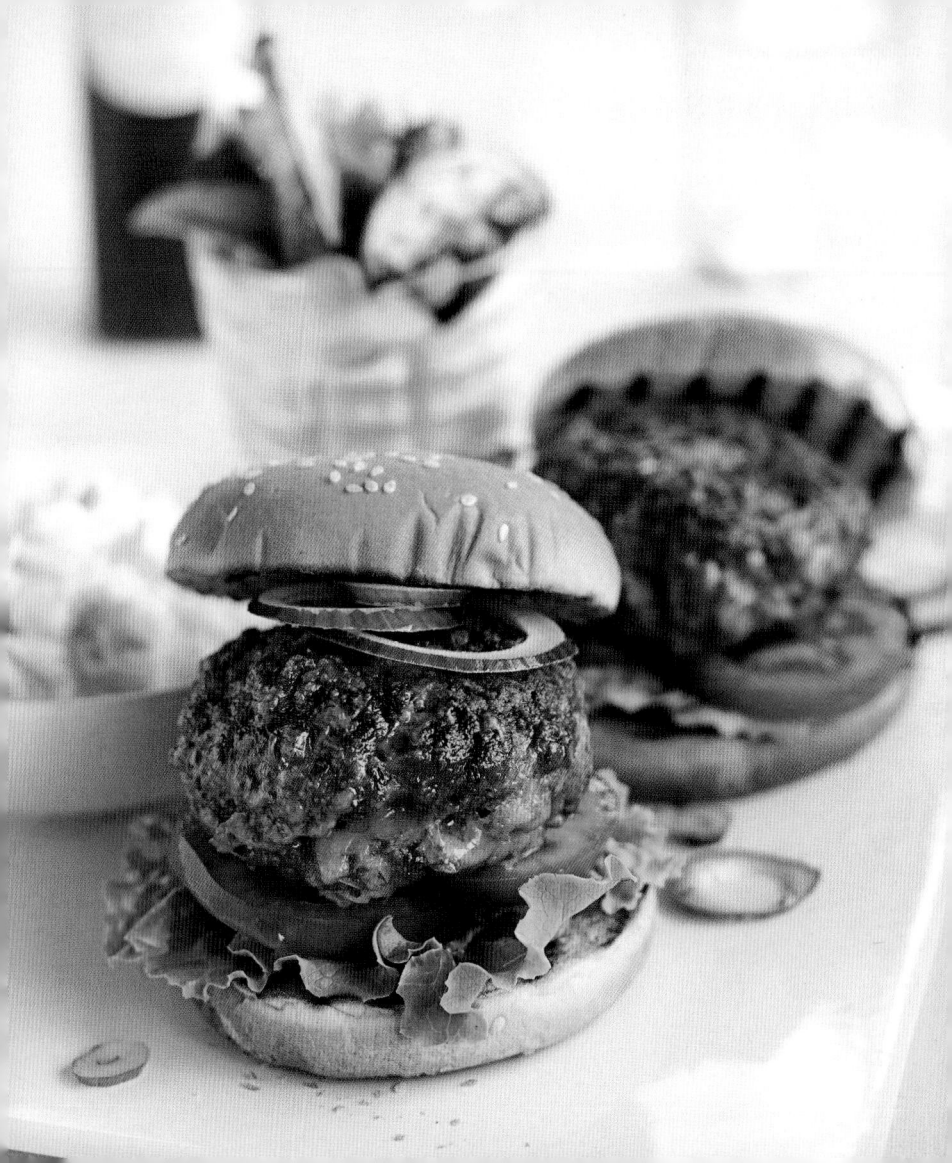

Steak, ale & mushroom pie

Who can resist a proper beef pie? Smoky bacon chunks, rich gravy, tender chunks of meat and lots of lovely veg.

TAKES 4 HOURS • SERVES 6

1kg/2lb 4oz braising steak, cut into
    very large chunks
2 onions, roughly chopped
2 carrots, chopped into large chunks
200g/7oz smoked bacon lardons
2 tbsp vegetable oil
300ml/½ pint dark ale
2 gluten-free beef stock cubes
small bunch each thyme, bay leaf and
    parsley, tied together
3 tbsp cornflour
200g/7oz chestnut mushrooms, halved

FOR THE PASTRY

600g/1lb 5oz gluten-free plain flour,
    plus extra for rolling
2 tsp xanthan gum
300g/10oz butter, diced, plus extra
    for greasing
3 eggs, beaten separately

1 Heat oven to 160C/140C fan/gas 3. Fry meat, onions, carrots and lardons in the oil in a casserole for 5 minutes. Add ale, stock, herbs and 400ml/14fl oz water; simmer. Cover and bake for 2 hours.
2 When the stew is done, return to the hob. Mix some sauce with cornflour to a paste, then whisk back into the stew and boil to thicken. Stir in the mushrooms.
3 Make pastry following method on p28, mixing in 4 tablespoons of water with two of the eggs to bring dough together.
4 Heat oven to 220C/200C fan/gas 7 with a baking sheet. Roll out two-thirds of the pastry to line a 24–28cm pie dish with an overhang. Add beef and veg with a slotted spoon. Spoon over some gravy. Brush pastry edges with third egg.
5 Roll out remaining pastry to cover the dish. Trim edges and crimp pastry to seal. Brush with more egg. Make a slit in the centre, sit on the baking sheet, then bake for 40 minutes until golden. Heat up leftover gravy to serve.

PER SERVING 1249 kcals, protein 51g, carbs 102g, fat 70g, sat fat 37g, fibre 4.5g, sugar 7g, salt 3.9g

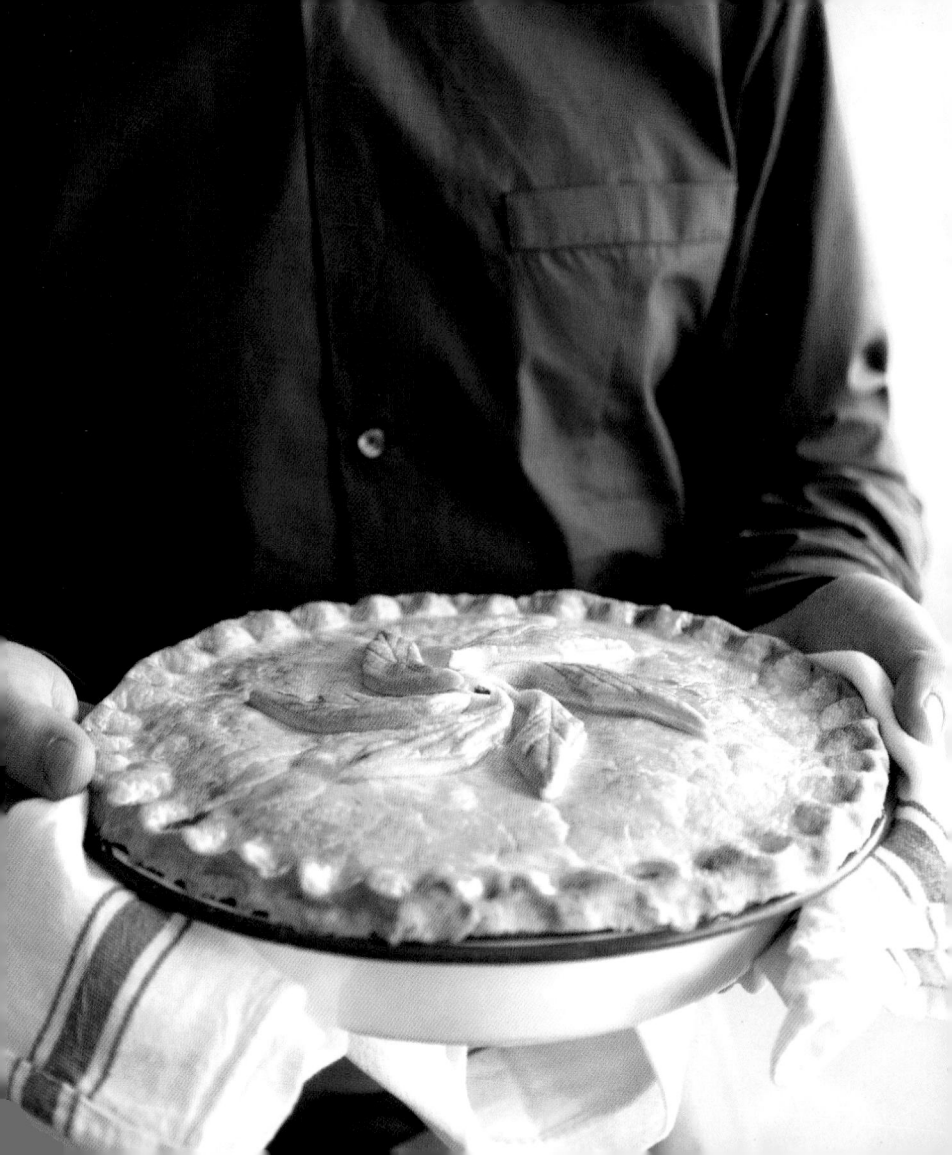

Sweet potato falafels with coleslaw

This low-fat supper is a great way to get veg into the kids – if you can't find gluten-free pitta bread simply serve with brown rice.

TAKES 1 HOUR 10 MINUTES

● **SERVES 4**

700g/1lb 9oz sweet potatoes
1 tsp ground cumin
2 garlic cloves, crushed
2 tsp ground coriander
handful coriander leaves, chopped
juice ½ lemon
100g/4oz gram flour
1 tbsp olive oil, for greasing
4 gluten-free pitta breads
4 tbsp reduced-fat houmous

FOR THE COLESLAW

2 tbsp red wine vinegar
1 tbsp golden caster sugar
1 small onion, finely sliced
1 medium carrot, grated
¼ each white and red cabbage, shredded

1 Heat oven to 200C/180C fan/gas 6. Microwave the sweet potatoes whole for 8–10 minutes until tender. Leave to cool a little, then peel. Put the potatoes, cumin, garlic, ground and fresh coriander, lemon juice and flour into a large bowl. Season, then mash until smooth. Using a tablespoon, shape the mix into 20 balls. Put on an oiled baking sheet, bake for around 15 minutes until the bases are golden brown, then flip over and bake for 15 minutes more until brown all over.

2 Meanwhile, stir together the vinegar and sugar for the coleslaw in a large bowl until the sugar has dissolved, toss through the onion, carrot and cabbage, then leave to marinate for 15 minutes.

3 To serve, toast the pittas, then split. Fill with the coleslaw, a dollop of houmous and the falafels.

PER SERVING 486 kcals, protein 16g, carbs 92g, fat 8g, sat fat 1g, fibre 14g, sugar 24g, salt 1.08g

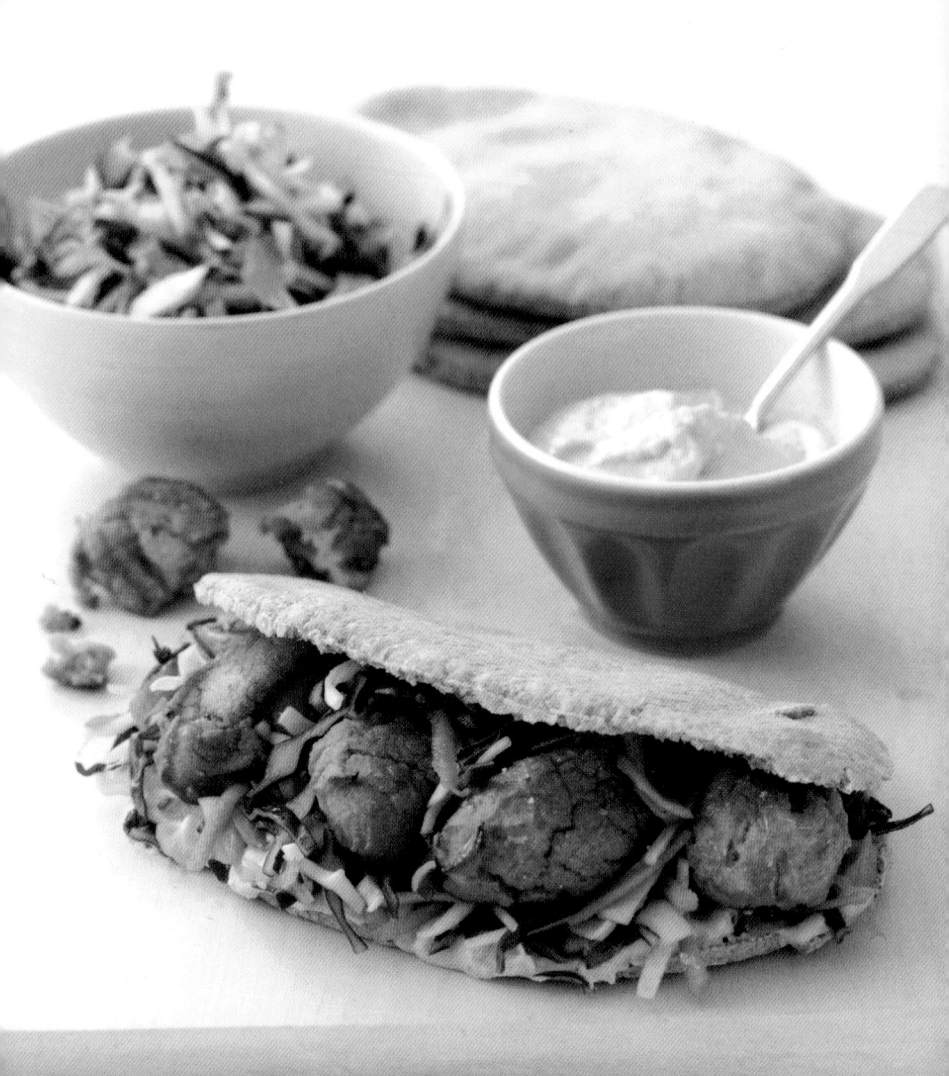

Crunchy chicken with noodle salad

If chillies are a bit fiery for your children leave them out and add a drizzle of sweet chilli sauce instead.

TAKES 30 MINUTES • SERVES 4

140g/5oz unsalted roasted peanuts

4 skinless chicken breasts, halved lengthways

1 egg, beaten lightly with a fork

85g/3oz dried soba or buckwheat noodles

1 cucumber, halved and sliced

small bunch mint, leaves picked and larger ones roughly chopped

zest and juice 2 limes, plus extra wedges to squeeze over

1–2 tsp sugar

1 red chilli, deseeded and finely sliced (optional)

1 Heat oven to 200C/180C fan/gas 6 and cover a baking sheet with baking parchment. Finely chop the peanuts in a food processor or by hand – you want large crumbs, not dust – then tip on to a plate.

2 Dip the chicken pieces in egg, then coat in the peanuts and put on the baking sheet. You can freeze the coated chicken pieces now for up to a month, defrost, then continue with recipe. Bake for 15–20 minutes until golden and cooked through.

3 Meanwhile, cook the noodles according to the pack instructions, drain, rinse under cold water until cool, then drain again. When the chicken is ready, use kitchen tongs or two forks to mix the noodles with the cucumber slices, mint, lime juice and zest, sugar, chilli, if using, and some seasoning. Serve immediately, topped with the crunchy chicken and lemon wedges alongside to squeeze over.

PER SERVING 483 kcals, protein 49g, carbs 24g, fat 22g, sat fat 5g, fibre 3g, sugar 5g, salt 0.70g

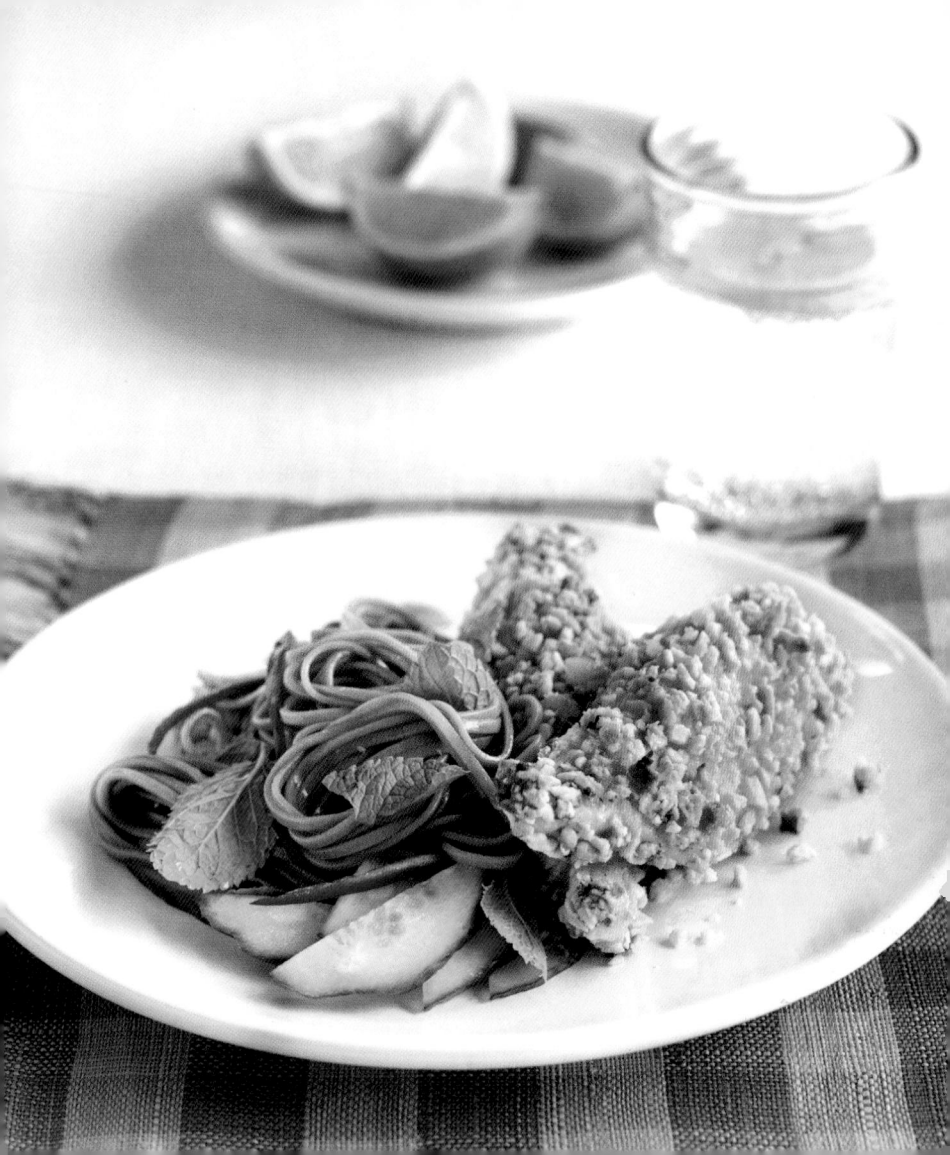

Toad in the hole

No one should have to miss out on toad in the hole – it's just too good! Equally tasty served with baked beans and tomato sauce, or gravy and veg.

TAKES 1 HOUR ● SERVES 4

12 gluten-free chipolata sausages
1 tbsp sunflower oil

FOR THE BATTER

140g/5oz gluten-free plain flour
50g/2oz cornflour
3 eggs
175ml/6fl oz semi-skimmed milk

1 Heat oven to 220C/200C fan/gas 7. Put the sausages in a 20 × 30cm roasting tin with the oil, then bake for 15 minutes until browned.

2 Meanwhile, make up the batter mix. Tip the flours into a bowl with ½ teaspoon salt, make a well in the middle and crack the eggs into it. Whisk it together, then slowly add the milk, whisking all the time until lump-free. Leave to stand until the sausages are nice and brown.

3 Carefully remove the sausages from the oven – watch because the fat will be sizzling hot, but if it isn't, put the tin on the hob for a few minutes until it is. Pour in the batter mix, transfer to the top shelf of the oven, then cook for 25–30 minutes, until risen and golden.

PER SERVING 472 kcals, protein 19g, carbs 37g, fat 29g, sat fat 9g, fibre 2g, sugar 5g, salt 2.34g

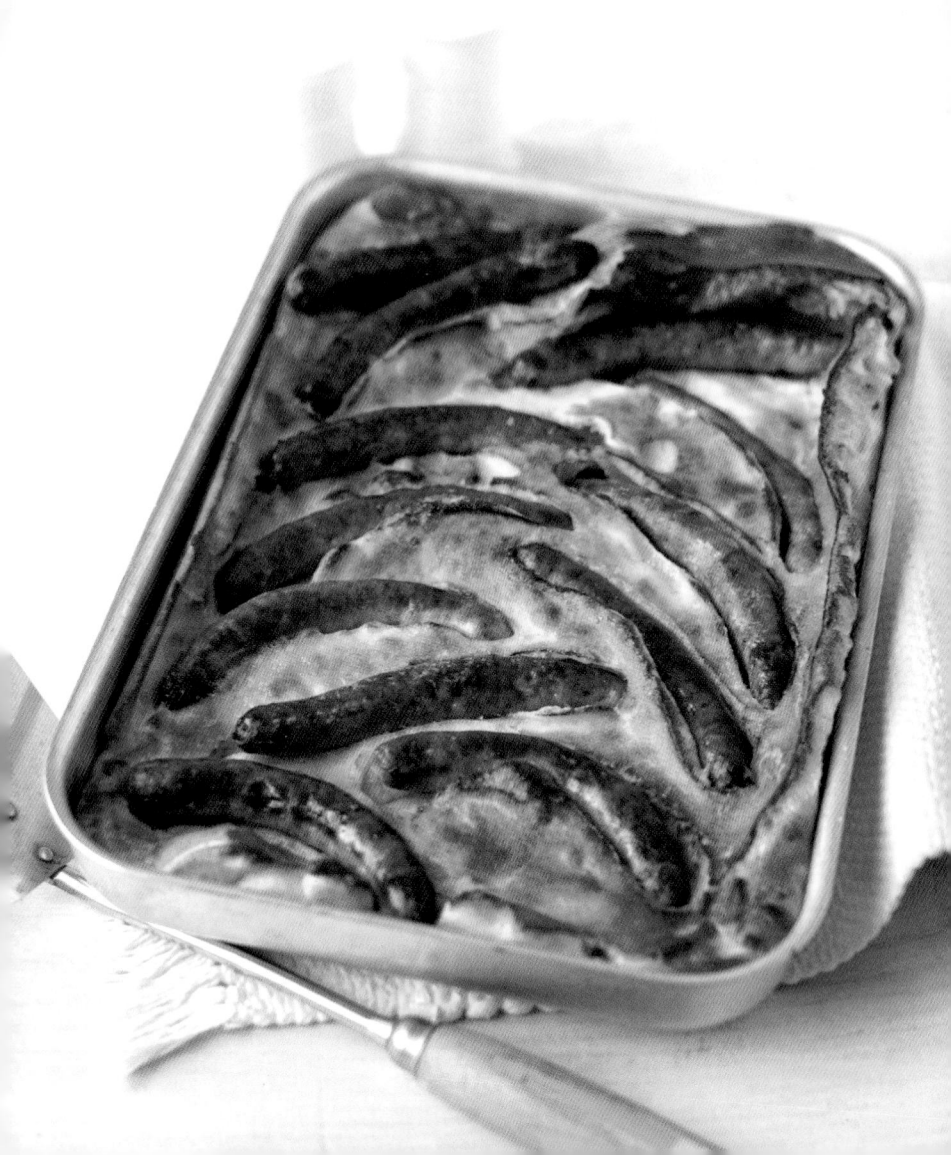

Crunchy fish goujons with skinny chips

No need for breadcrumbs for these kids' favourites – they're cleverly coated in crispy gluten-free cornflakes.

TAKES 15 MINUTES • SERVES 4

2 large potatoes, cut into skinny chips
2 tbsp olive oil
450g/1lb chunky fish fillets cut into
    finger-sized strips
2 eggs, beaten
140g/5oz gluten-free cornflakes,
    crushed into crumbs
lemon wedges, to garnish
tartare sauce or tomato ketchup,
    to serve

1 Heat oven to 200C/180C fan/gas 6. Put the chips on a baking sheet, toss with oil and season. Cook for 20 minutes on the top shelf.

2 Dip the fish strips in the egg and then the cornflakes. Lay on a wire rack over a baking sheet. Transfer the chips to a lower shelf, then cook the fish above for 15 minutes, turning halfway through, until crisp and golden.

3 Serve the goujons and chips with tartare sauce or tomato ketchup and lemon wedges on the side.

PER SERVING 382 kcals, protein 27g, carbs 49g, fat 10g, sat fat 2g, fibre 2g, sugar 4g, salt 1.30g

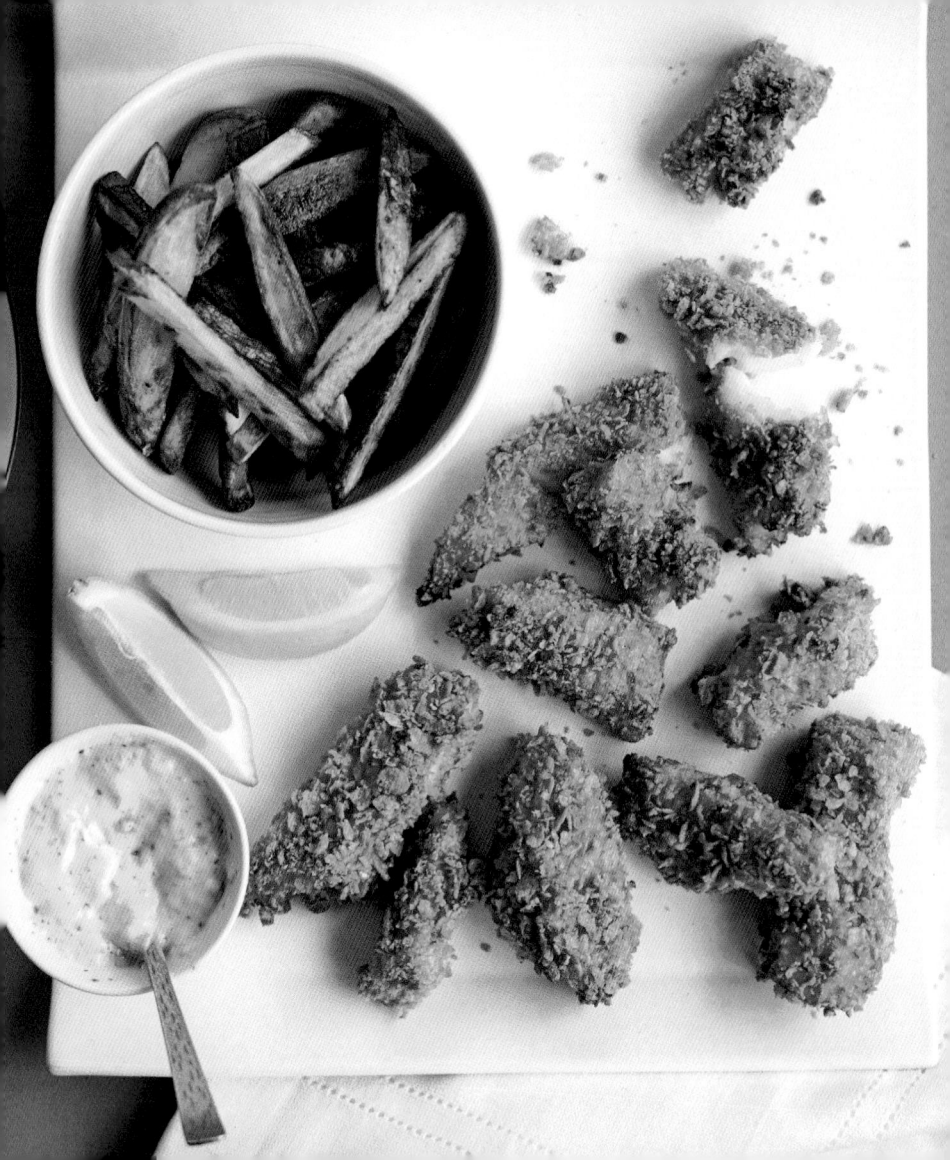

Tuna arrabbiata pasta gratin

This is a great family supper that the whole family will enjoy. If the kids don't like tuna, add some bacon bits instead.

TAKES 30 MINUTES • SERVES 4

1 tsp olive oil

1 red and 1 yellow pepper, deseeded
    and sliced

2 garlic cloves, crushed

pinch crushed dried chillies

2 × 400g cans chopped tomatoes

50g/2oz mixed pitted olives, whole or
    roughly chopped (optional)

pinch caster sugar

250g/9oz gluten-free pasta shapes

2 × 200g cans tuna steak in spring
    water, drained and flaked

25g/1oz gluten-free bread, whizzed
    into crumbs

2 tbsp grated Parmesan

1 Heat the oil in a large pan and fry the peppers for about 5 minutes until starting to caramelise. Add the garlic and chillies, cook for 30 seconds, then tip in the tomatoes and olives (if using). Season, add the sugar, bring to the boil, then simmer the sauce, uncovered, for 10 minutes.

2 Meanwhile, cook the pasta according to the pack instructions. Heat the grill. Drain the pasta and mix into the tomato sauce, along with the tuna. Tip into a large ovenproof dish. Mix the breadcrumbs and Parmesan together, and scatter over the top. Grill for 3–4 minutes or until the topping is crisp and golden. Serve immediately.

PER SERVING 365 kcals, protein 30g, carbs 54g, fat 5g, sat fat 1g, fibre 9g, sugar 11g, salt 0.75g

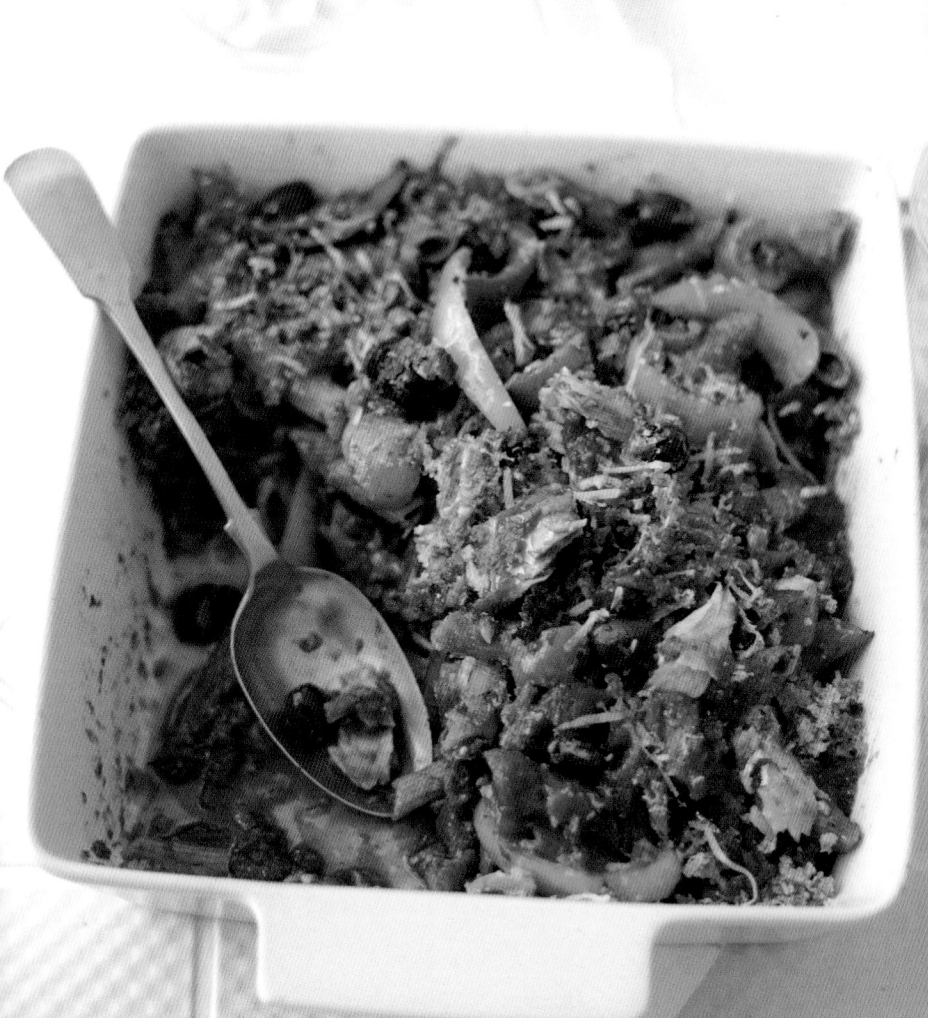

Nutty chicken curry

This mild, creamy dish is loosely based on an African-style curry that often has peanuts in the sauce. Using peanut butter might seem odd, but it's a delicious cheat!

TAKES 20 MINUTES ● SERVES 4

1 large red chilli, deseeded
½ finger-length piece root ginger, roughly chopped
1 fat garlic clove
small bunch coriander, stalks roughly chopped
1 tbsp sunflower oil
4 boneless skinless chicken breasts, cut into chunks
5 tbsp gluten-free peanut butter
150ml/¼ pint gluten-free chicken stock
200g tub thick Greek yogurt
rice or mashed sweet potato, to serve

1 Finely slice and set aside a quarter of the chilli, then put the rest in a food processor with the ginger, garlic, coriander stalks and one-third of the leaves. Whizz to a rough paste with a splash of water, if needed.

2 Heat the oil in a frying pan, then quickly brown the chicken chunks for 1 minute. Stir in the paste for another minute, then add the peanut butter, stock and yogurt. When the sauce is gently bubbling, cook for 10 minutes until the chicken is just cooked through and the sauce thickened.

3 Stir in most of the remaining coriander leaves, then scatter the rest on top with the reserved sliced chilli. Eat with rice or mashed sweet potato.

PER SERVING 358 kcals, protein 43g, carbs 4g, fat 19g, sat fat 6g, fibre 1g, sugar 3g, salt 0.66g

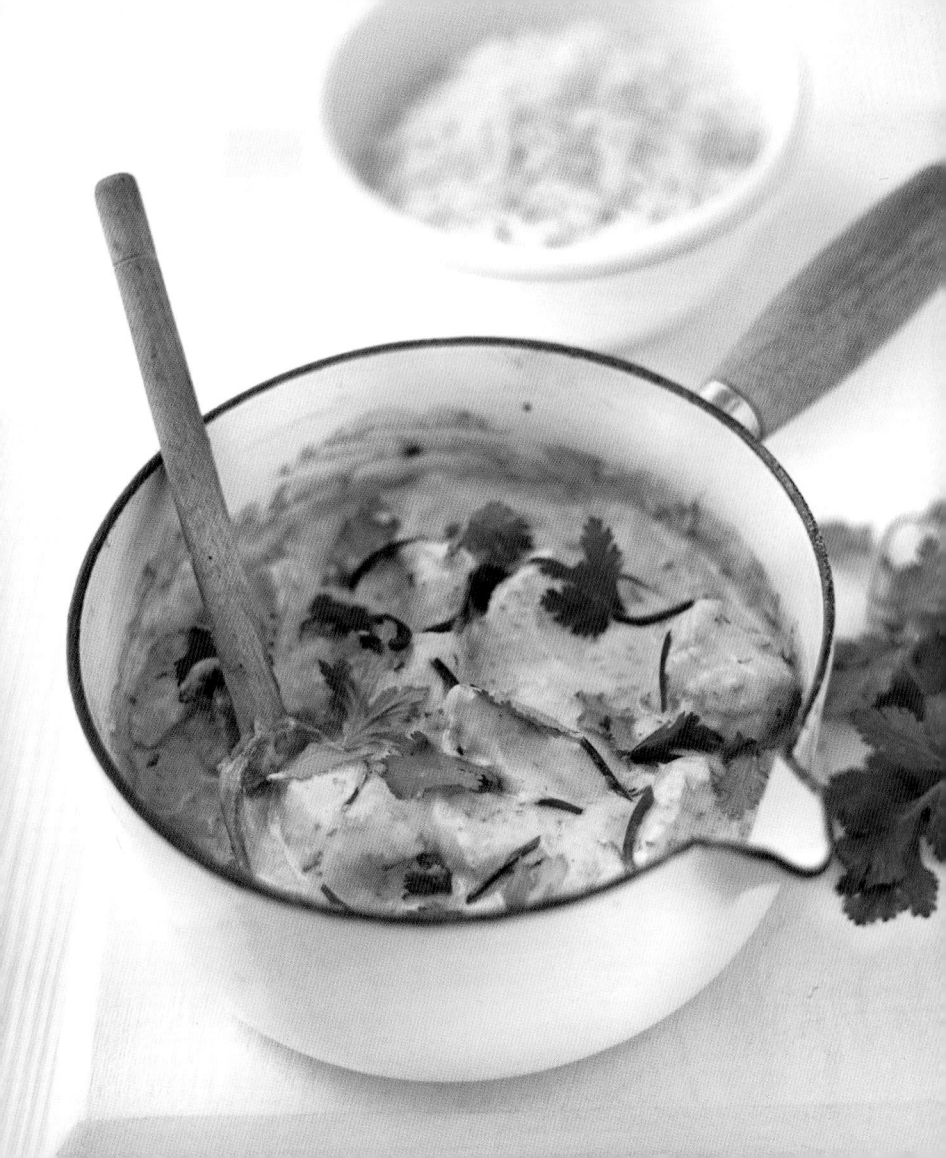

Mushroom & chickpea burgers

Ready-made gluten-free veggie burgers are hard to find, and definitely not as tasty as these low-fat versions.

TAKES 30 MINUTES • SERVES 4

1 tbsp olive oil

250g/9oz chestnut mushrooms, finely chopped

2 garlic cloves, crushed

1 bunch spring onions, sliced

1 tbsp medium gluten-free curry powder

zest and juice ½ lemon

400g can chickpeas, rinsed and drained

85g/3oz gluten-free wholemeal bread, whizzed into crumbs

6 tbsp 0% thick Greek yogurt

pinch ground cumin

2 gluten-free rolls, toasted and halved

2 plum tomatoes, sliced

handful rocket leaves

1 Heat 1 teaspoon of the oil in a non-stick frying pan and cook the mushrooms, garlic and spring onions for 5 minutes. Mix in the curry powder, lemon zest and juice, and cook for 2 minutes or until the mixture looks quite dry. Tip out on to a plate to cool slightly.

2 Use a potato masher or fork to mash the chickpeas in a bowl, leaving a few chunky pieces. Add the mushroom mix and the crumbs, then shape into four patties. Fry in the remaining oil for 3–4 minutes on each side until crisp and browned.

3 Mix the yogurt with the cumin. Put half a roll on each plate, then spread with the yogurt. Top with the burgers, a few slices of tomato and a little rocket.

PER SERVING 271 kcals, protein 15g, carbs 40g, fat 7g, sat fat 1g, fibre 6g, sugar 4g, salt 1.13g

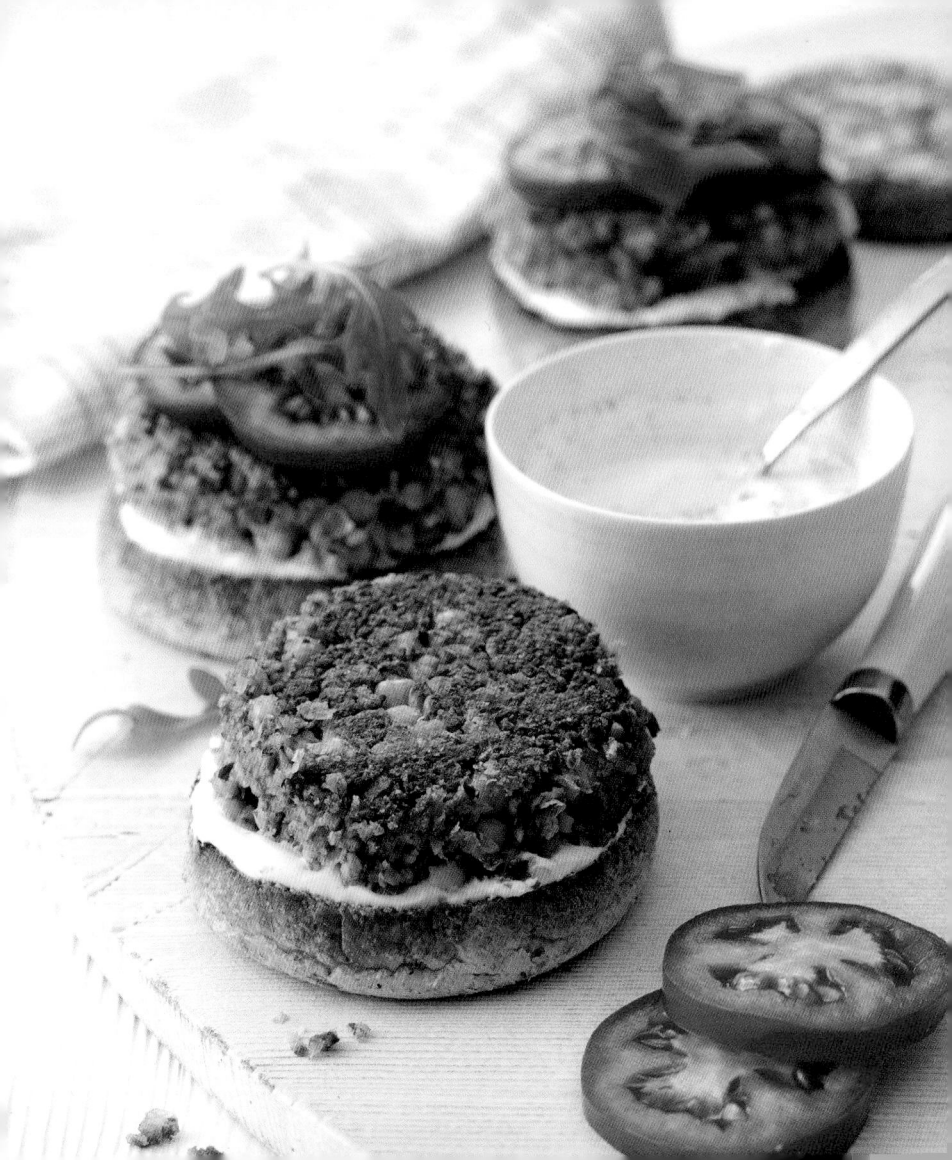

Cheat's chicken Kiev

Making real chicken Kievs is a labour of love, so this clever traybake has all the classic flavours involved, but none of the hard work!

TAKES 40 MINUTES ● MAKES 4

6 garlic cloves, 2 peeled
small bunch flat-leaf parsley
4 tsp olive oil
85g/3oz gluten-free bread, whizzed
   into crumbs
4 skinless boneless chicken breasts
4 tbsp garlic & herb soft cheese

1 Heat oven to 200C/180C fan/gas 6. Whizz together the 2 peeled garlic cloves, parsley and 1 teaspoon of the olive oil in a food processor. Add the breadcrumbs and some seasoning before pulsing briefly to mix. Tip on to a plate.

2 Cut a slit (roughly thumb-length) in the side of each chicken breast, at the plump end. Spoon a quarter of the soft cheese into each hole and press the edges together to seal. Rub 2 teaspoons oil over all the chicken breasts before pressing the herby crumbs onto them.

3 Put the coated chicken in a shallow roasting tin. Scatter round the remaining unpeeled garlic cloves and drizzle with the rest of the oil. Bake for 20–25 minutes until the chicken is cooked and the crumbs are crisp and golden. Squeeze out the soft, roasted garlic from the skins and serve with the chicken.

PER KIEV 327 kcals, protein 38g, carbs 18g, fat 12g, sat fat 5g, fibre 1g, sugar 1g, salt 0.78g

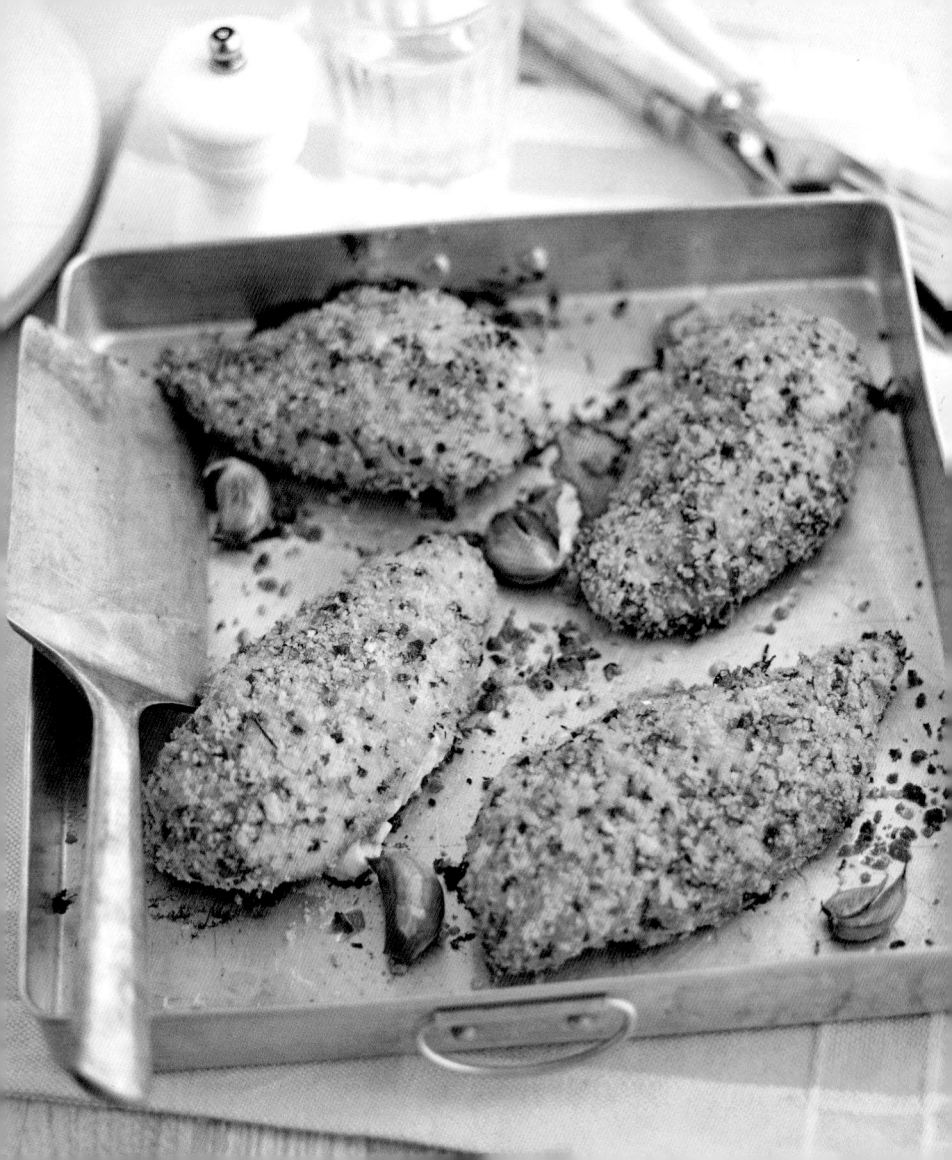

Coconut noodle & vegetable soup

Gluten-free rice noodles are a great alternative to egg noodles in Thai and Chinese recipes.

TAKES 25 MINUTES • SERVES 4

1–2 tbsp gluten-free Thai green curry paste
1 tsp groundnut oil
700ml/1¼ pints gluten-free vegetable stock
300ml/½ pint reduced-fat coconut milk
200g/7oz thick rice noodles
200g/7oz chestnut mushrooms, sliced
140g/5oz sugar snap peas, halved
100g/4oz beansprouts
1½ tbsp Thai fish sauce
juice 1 lime
3 spring onions, shredded, to garnish
few mint and coriander leaves, to serve

1 Put a large pan over a medium heat. Cook the curry paste in the oil for 1 minute until it starts to release its aroma. Pour in the stock and coconut milk, and bring to the boil. Reduce the heat to a simmer and stir in the noodles. Simmer for 7 minutes, then stir in the mushrooms and sugar snaps. Cook for 3 minutes more, then add the beansprouts, fish sauce and lime juice. Remove the pan from the heat.
2 Ladle the noodles and soup into bowls, then scatter with spring onions, mint and coriander to serve.

PER SERVING 296 kcals, protein 7g, carbs 48g, fat 10g, sat fat 7g, fibre 3g, sugar 5g, salt 1.97g

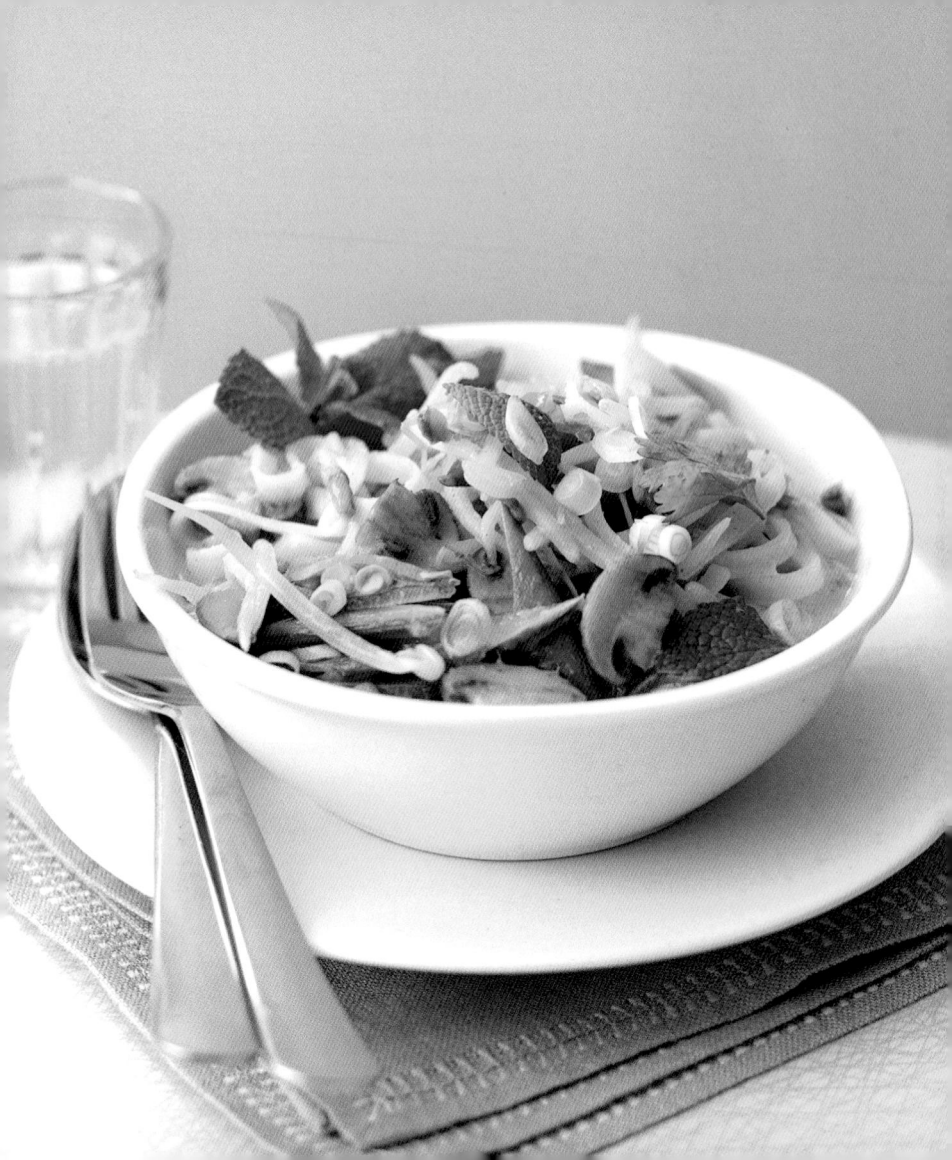

Pork & quinoa-stuffed peppers

Peppers are often much better value bought in big multi-packs of mixed colours.
If you're not so keen on quinoa, you could always use rice instead.

TAKES 40 MINUTES ● SERVES 4

4 peppers, halved, deseeded and cores
  removed
200g/7oz minced pork
1 garlic clove, crushed
2 tsp ground cumin
1 tsp paprika
50g/2oz quinoa
250ml/9fl oz gluten-free vegetable
  stock
½ small bunch parsley, chopped
4 tbsp 0% thick Greek yogurt, to serve

1 Put the peppers, cut-side down, on a plate and microwave on High for 4 minutes until cooked through (but not so soft that they collapse). If they need longer, microwave for 1 minute more and repeat until done.
2 Put the pork in a cold frying pan and turn on the heat. Fry, breaking up any lumps, until it starts to brown. Stir in the garlic and spices for 1 minute, then add the quinoa and stock. Cover and simmer for 10–15 minutes until the quinoa is soft.
3 Heat the grill. Stir half the parsley into the quinoa, then stuff into the peppers on a baking sheet. Grill to crisp, sprinkle over most of the remaining parsley, then serve with the yogurt mixed with the rest of the parsley.

PER SERVING 192 kcals, protein 16g, carbs 18g, fat 7g, sat fat 2g, fibre 4g, sugar 11g, salt 0.3g

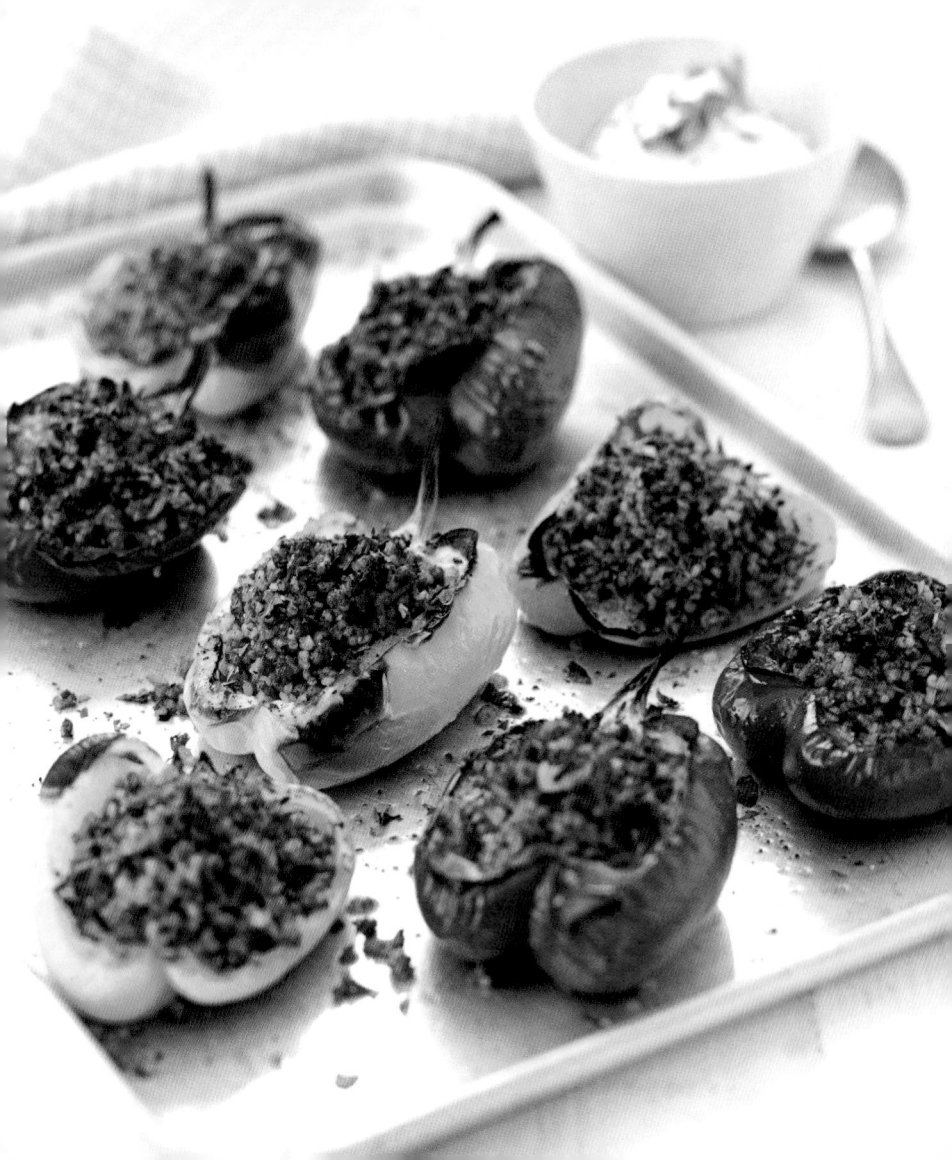

Mumbai potato wraps with minted yogurt relish

This is a great storecupboard supper – you'll probably have most of the ingredients already.

TAKES 50 MINUTES • **SERVES 4**

2 tsp sunflower oil
1 onion, sliced
2 tbsp medium gluten-free curry
    powder
400g can chopped tomatoes
750g/1lb 10oz potatoes, diced
2 tbsp spiced mango chutney, plus
    extra to serve (optional)
100g/4oz low-fat natural yogurt
1 tsp mint sauce from a jar
8 gluten-free chapatis or wraps
coriander sprigs, to garnish

1 Heat the sunflower oil in a large pan and fry the onion for 6–8 minutes until golden and soft. Stir in 1½ tablespoons of the curry powder, cook for 30 seconds, then add the tomatoes and some seasoning. Simmer the sauce, uncovered, for 15 minutes.

2 Meanwhile, add the potatoes and the remaining curry powder to a pan of boiling salted water. Cook for 6–8 minutes until just tender. Drain, reserving 100ml/3½fl oz of the liquid. Add the drained potatoes and reserved liquid to the tomato sauce along with the mango chutney. Heat through.

3 Meanwhile, mix together the yogurt and mint sauce, and warm the chapatis or wraps according to the pack instructions.

4 To serve, spoon some of the potatoes on to a chapati or wrap and top with a few sprigs of coriander. Drizzle with the minted yogurt relish, adding extra mango chutney if you wish, then roll up and eat.

PER SERVING 230 kcals, protein 8g, carbs 45g, fat 4g, sat fat 1g, fibre 6g, sugar 10g, salt 0.57g

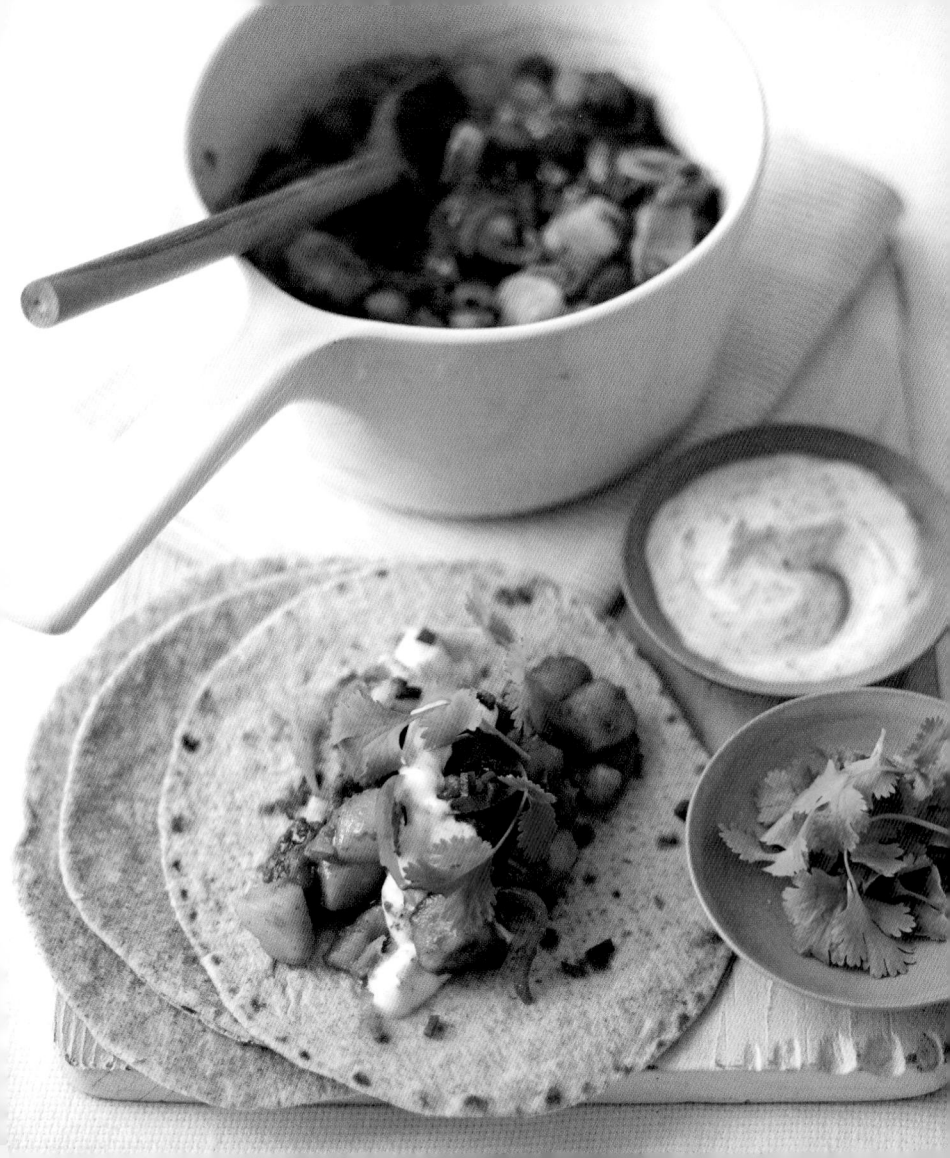

Vietnamese prawn salad

This no-cook salad is low fat, so why not make double of it and save some for lunchboxes the following day?

TAKES 20 MINUTES • SERVES 2

FOR THE DRESSING

1 small garlic clove, finely chopped
1 tbsp sweet chilli sauce
1 tbsp golden caster sugar
juice 2 limes

FOR THE SALAD

250g/9oz thin rice noodles
150g pack cooked tiger prawns, halved along their spine
½ cucumber, peeled, deseeded and cut into matchsticks
1 carrot, cut into matchsticks or grated
6 spring onions, shredded
handful coriander and/or mint leaves
1 tbsp roasted peanuts, chopped

1 To make the dressing, mash the garlic, chilli and sugar using a pestle and mortar. Add the lime juice and 3 tablespoons water, and stir together. Set aside.

2 Get the kettle on, put the noodles into a bowl, then cover with boiling water. Leave to stand for 10 minutes until tender, then drain and divide between two bowls.

3 Mix the prawns and veg together, and divide between the bowls, too. Finish by topping each salad with the herbs and peanuts, then pour over the dressing to serve.

PER SERVING 579 kcals, protein 27g, carbs 117g, fat 4g, sat fat 1g, fibre 2g, sugar 14g, salt 1.66g

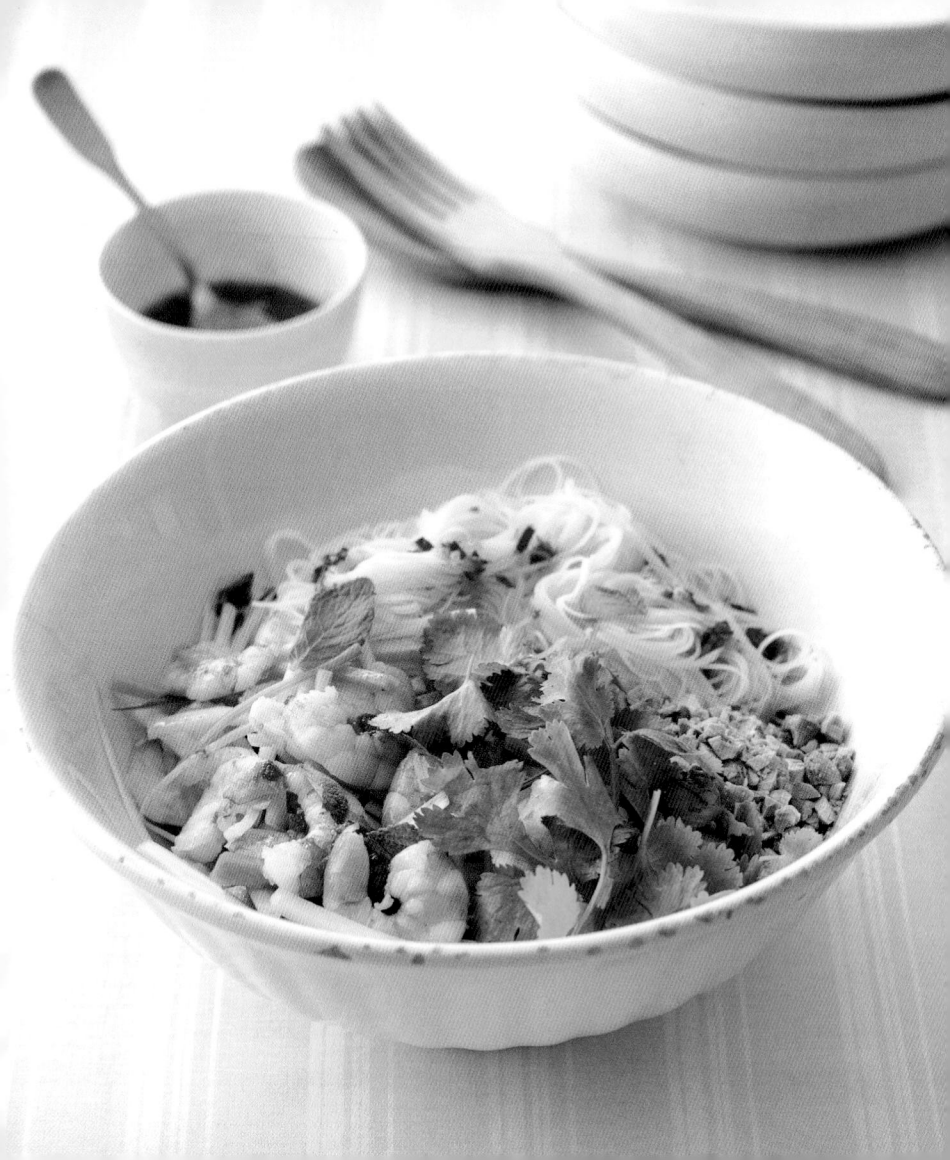

Spiced pork & potato pie

This French-Canadian speciality, known as Tourtière, is traditionally served at Christmas, but eaten with salad or veg it makes a popular supper all year round.

TAKES 55 MINUTES, PLUS CHILLING

● **SERVES 6**

1 medium potato, cut into chunks
1 tsp sunflower oil
500g pack lean minced pork
1 onion, finely chopped
1 garlic clove, chopped
¼ tsp each ground cinnamon, allspice
  and nutmeg
100ml/3½fl oz gluten-free chicken
  stock

FOR THE PASTRY

300g/10oz gluten-free plain flour
1 tsp xanthan gum
140g/5oz butter, diced
2 eggs, beaten separately

1 Heat oven to 200C/180C fan/gas 6. Boil the potato until tender, drain and mash, then leave to cool. Heat the oil in a non-stick pan, add the mince and onion, and quickly fry until browned. Mix in the garlic, spices, stock, plenty of pepper and a little salt. Remove from the heat, stir into the potato and cool.

2 Make the pastry following the method on p28.

3 Roll out half the pastry and line the base of a 20–23cm pie plate or flan tin. Fill with the pork mixture and brush the edges of the pastry with water. Roll out the remaining dough and cover the pie. Press the edges to seal, trimming off the excess. Prick the top of the pastry case to allow steam to escape and glaze the top with the remaining beaten egg.

4 Bake for 30 minutes until the pastry is crisp and golden. Serve cut into wedges. Any leftovers are good cold for lunch the next day, served with a selection of pickles.

PER SERVING 466 kcals, protein 26g, carbs 37g, fat 25g, sat fat 9g, fibre 2g, sugar 2g, salt 0.9g

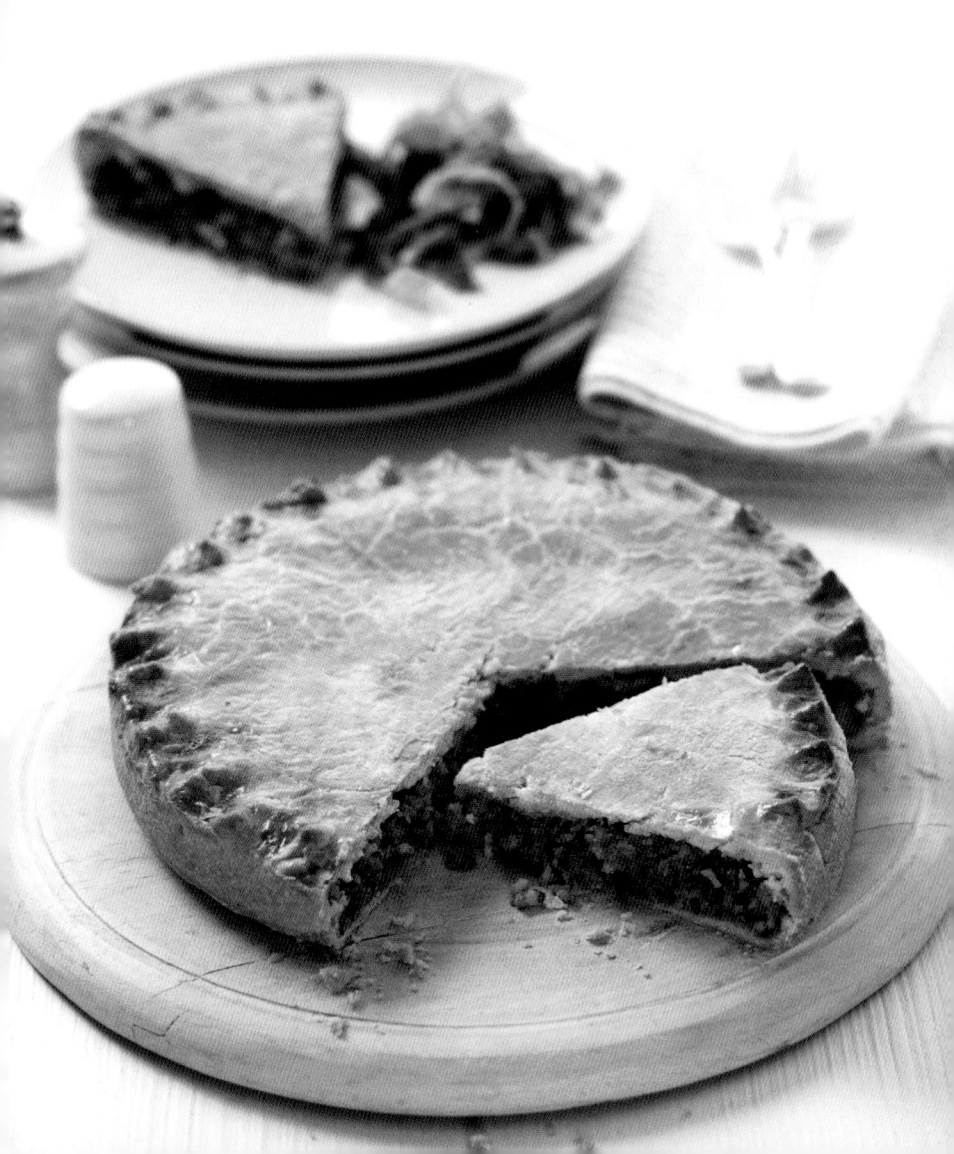

Polenta tart with sausage & broccoli

You may have tried wet polenta as a good alternative to mash, but if you let it set until firm it makes a great fuss-free tart or pizza base.

TAKES 40 MINUTES ● SERVES 4

1 litre/1¾ pints gluten-free vegetable stock
200g/7oz instant polenta
50g/2oz Parmesan, grated
140g/5oz thin-stemmed broccoli
200g/7oz ready-grated mozzarella
100g/4oz semi-dried tomatoes
1 garlic clove, chopped
4 gluten-free Italian pork sausages, skins removed and split into bite-sized chunks

1 Heat oven to 190C/170C fan/gas 5. In a large pan, bring the stock to the boil. Slowly pour in the polenta, a little at a time, until completely absorbed. Lower the heat, stir quickly for 5 minutes, then remove from the heat altogether. Stir in 1 tablespoon of the Parmesan and some seasoning, then spread the polenta out on a large parchment-lined baking sheet, so that it's 2–3cm/¾–1¼in thick.

2 Cook the broccoli in salted water for 2 minutes, drain, then rinse under cold water.

3 Sprinkle the mozzarella and remaining Parmesan over the polenta, then top with the tomatoes, garlic, broccoli and sausages. Bake for 20 minutes until the sausages are browned and the sides of the polenta are crisp.

PER SERVING 703 kcals, protein 29g, carbs 44g, fat 45g, sat fat 17g, fibre 3g, sugar 4g, salt 3.2g

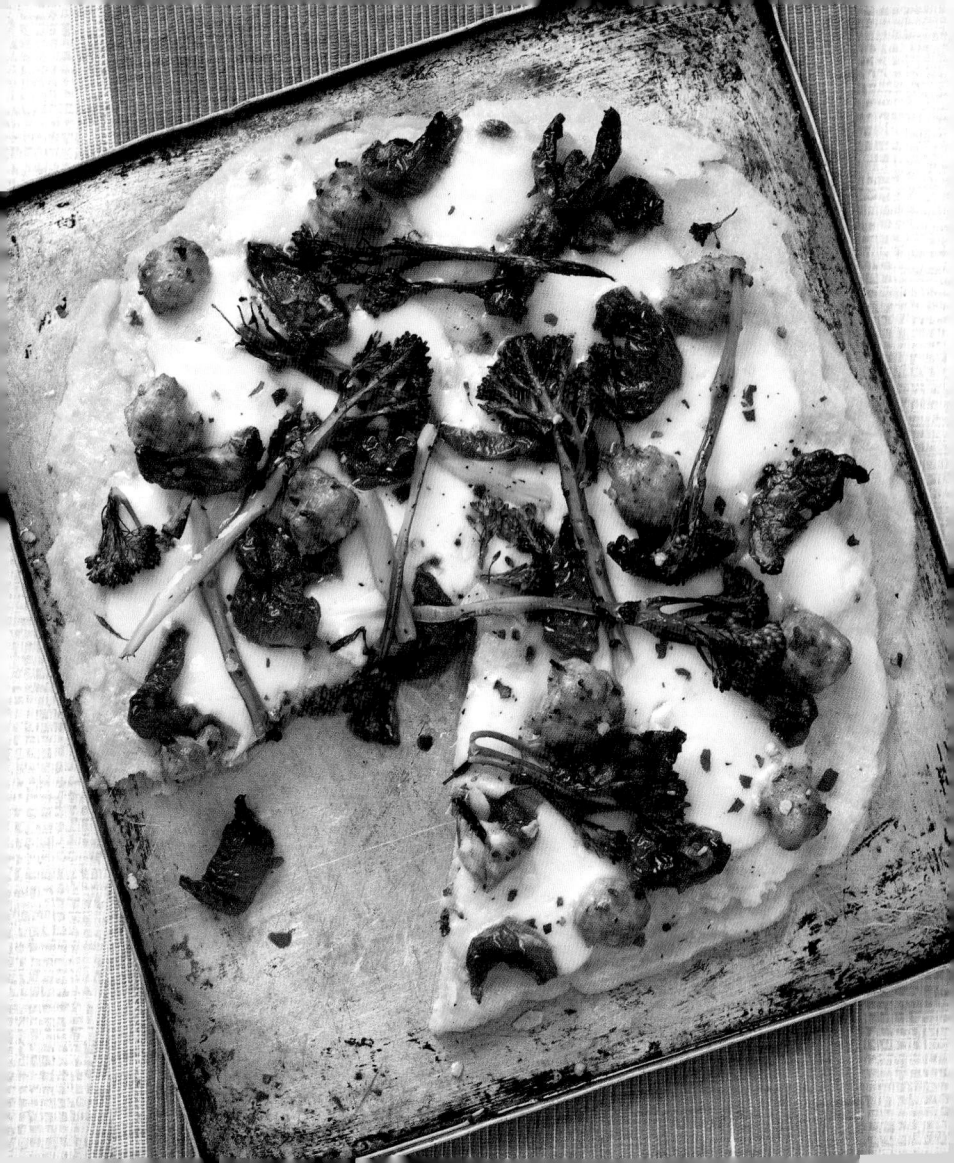

Spice crunch chicken with guacamole salad

A fun alternative to chicken nuggets, corn tortillas add an extra crunch. Serve this with a fresh chunky salad, or with cheesy mash and sweetcorn, if the kids prefer.

TAKES 20 MINUTES • SERVES 4

4 skinless chicken breasts
200g bag gluten-free tortilla chips
1½ tsp mild chilli powder
1 egg, beaten
2 avocados
4 tomatoes
½ red onion
juice 1 lime

1 Heat oven to 220C/200C fan/gas 7. Cover a baking sheet with parchment. Lay each chicken breast flat on a board, then halve through the middle so you get two thin breast-sized pieces from each.

2 Bash 85g/3oz of the tortillas into rough crumbs and small flakes, then tip into a shallow bowl with 1 teaspoon of the chilli powder and some salt. Mix well. Dip each piece of chicken into some of the beaten egg. Mix the remaining egg into the tortilla crumbs. Now dip each chicken piece into the crumbs so you have a patchy crust.

3 Roast on the baking sheet for 12 minutes until the chicken is cooked through. Cut the avocados and tomatoes for the guacamole into chunks and thinly slice the onion. Whisk the remaining chilli powder and some seasoning into the lime juice, then mix through the salad.

4 Serve 2 crispy chicken pieces per person with a spoonful of guacamole salad and a handful of the remaining tortillas.

PER SERVING 555 kcals, protein 42g, carbs 36g, fat 28g, sat fat 3g, fibre 6g, sugar 4g, salt 1.44g

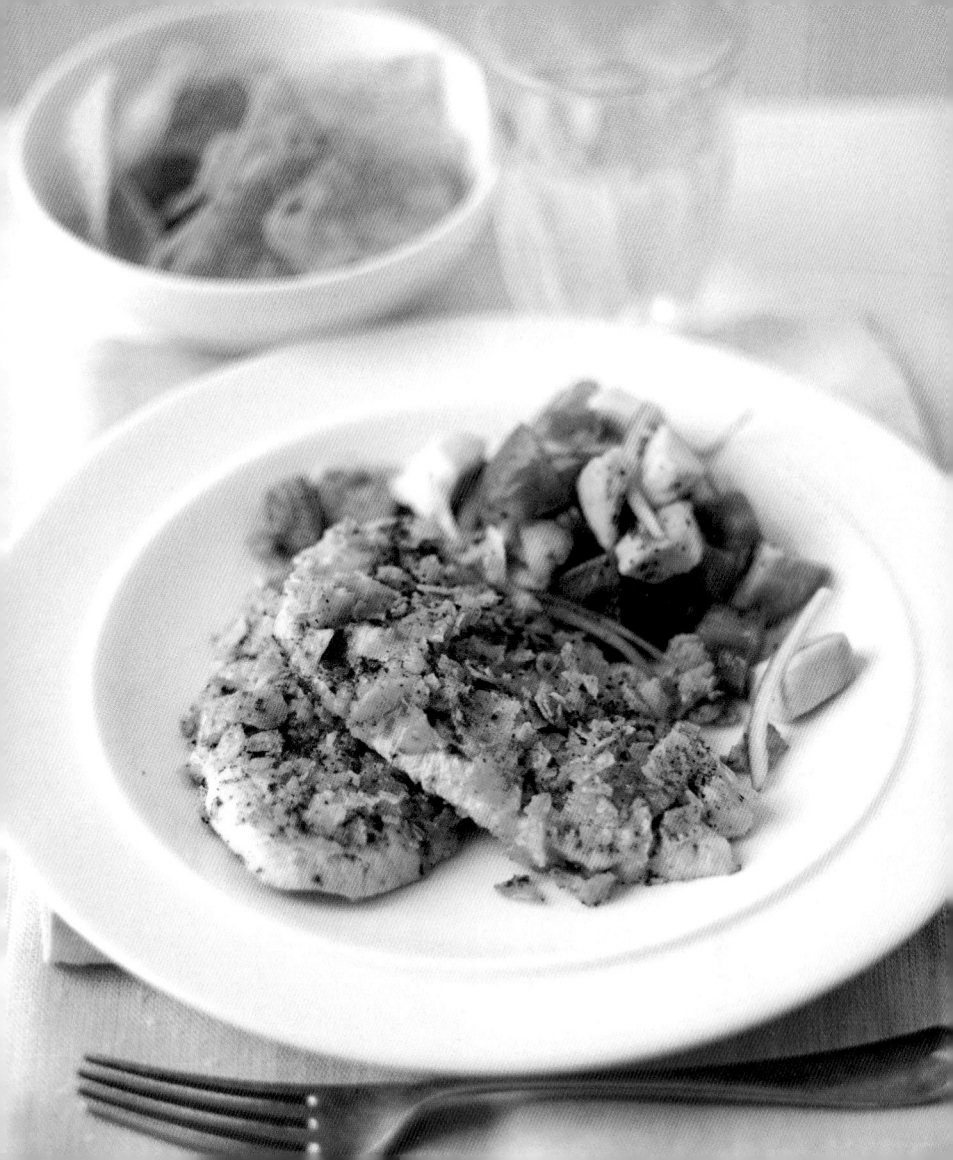

Full English pizza

This is a fun supper that kids of all ages will love – and can lend a hand to prepare too.

TAKES 40 MINUTES, PLUS RISING

● **SERVES 4**

6 tbsp passata

140g/5oz mushrooms, sliced

4 gluten-free pork sausages, skinned and quartered

8 streaky bacon rashers, halved

4 medium eggs

FOR THE DOUGH

450g/1lb gluten-free plain flour, plus extra for rolling

2 tsp xanthan gum

2 tsp caster sugar

1 × 7g sachet fast-action dried yeast

2 eggs, beaten

6 tbsp olive oil, plus extra for greasing

1 For the dough, mix the flour, gum, sugar, yeast and 1 teaspoon salt in a bowl. Make a well in the centre and add the eggs, oil and 250ml/9fl oz hand-warm water, and stir in with a wooden spoon to a sticky dough. Knead for 5 minutes on a lightly floured surface then sit in an oiled bowl, cover with a clean tea towel and leave somewhere warm-ish to rise for 30 minutes.

2 Heat oven to 220C/200C fan/gas 7. On a lightly floured surface, roll out the dough to fit a lightly oiled 30 × 40cm baking sheet, or two smaller trays. Spread the passata over the base and dot over the mushrooms. Sit the sausages and bacon in a small roasting tin and cook with the pizza for 20 minutes at the top of the oven.

3 Remove the pizza from the oven, dot over the sausages and bacon, and crack the eggs on. Return to the oven and cook for 5 minutes more, or longer depending how well-cooked you like your eggs.

PER SERVING 946 kcals, protein 28g, carbs 99g, fat 48g, sat fat 13g, fibre 3g, sugar 5g, salt 4.1g

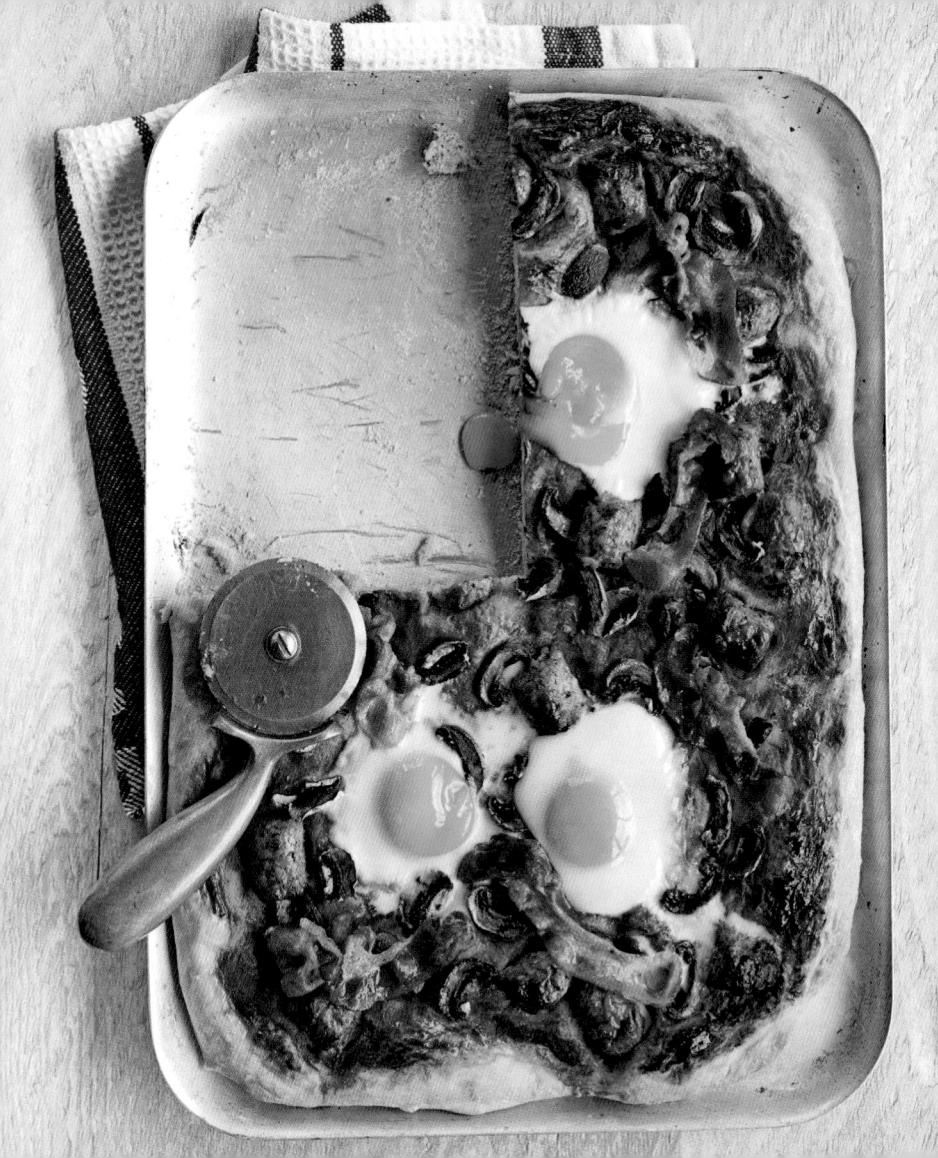

Fruit & nut granola

Fancy cereals can be really expensive and seem to disappear in just a few breakfasts. Make your own and you can decide exactly what to put in it.

TAKES 35 MINUTES • SERVES 14

1 tbsp vegetable oil
100ml/4fl oz clear honey
50ml/2fl oz maple syrup
500g/1lb 2oz gluten-free oats
100g/4oz flaked almonds
50g/2oz pine nuts
100g/4oz gluten-free puffed rice
2 tsp sesame seeds
50g/2oz each sultanas and raisins
85g/3oz each dried cranberries, dried
 cherries, chopped dried dates and
 chopped dried apricots
50g/2oz dried coconut shavings or
 desiccated coconut

1 Heat oven to 160C/140C fan/gas 3. Heat the oil, honey and maple syrup together in a pan. Mix the oats, almonds, pine nuts, puffed rice and sesame seeds in a large mixing bowl. Pour over the honey mix, stir well to coat, then tip on to a large baking tin. Bake for 15 minutes until everything is golden and crisp.

2 Take the tin from the oven, leave to cool, then break up any big clumps. Mix together with the dried fruit and coconut shavings. Store in a sealed jar and enjoy over the next 2 weeks.

PER SERVING 374 kcals, protein 8g, carbs 62g, fat 13g, sat fat 3g, fibre 5g, sugar 31g, salt 0.17g

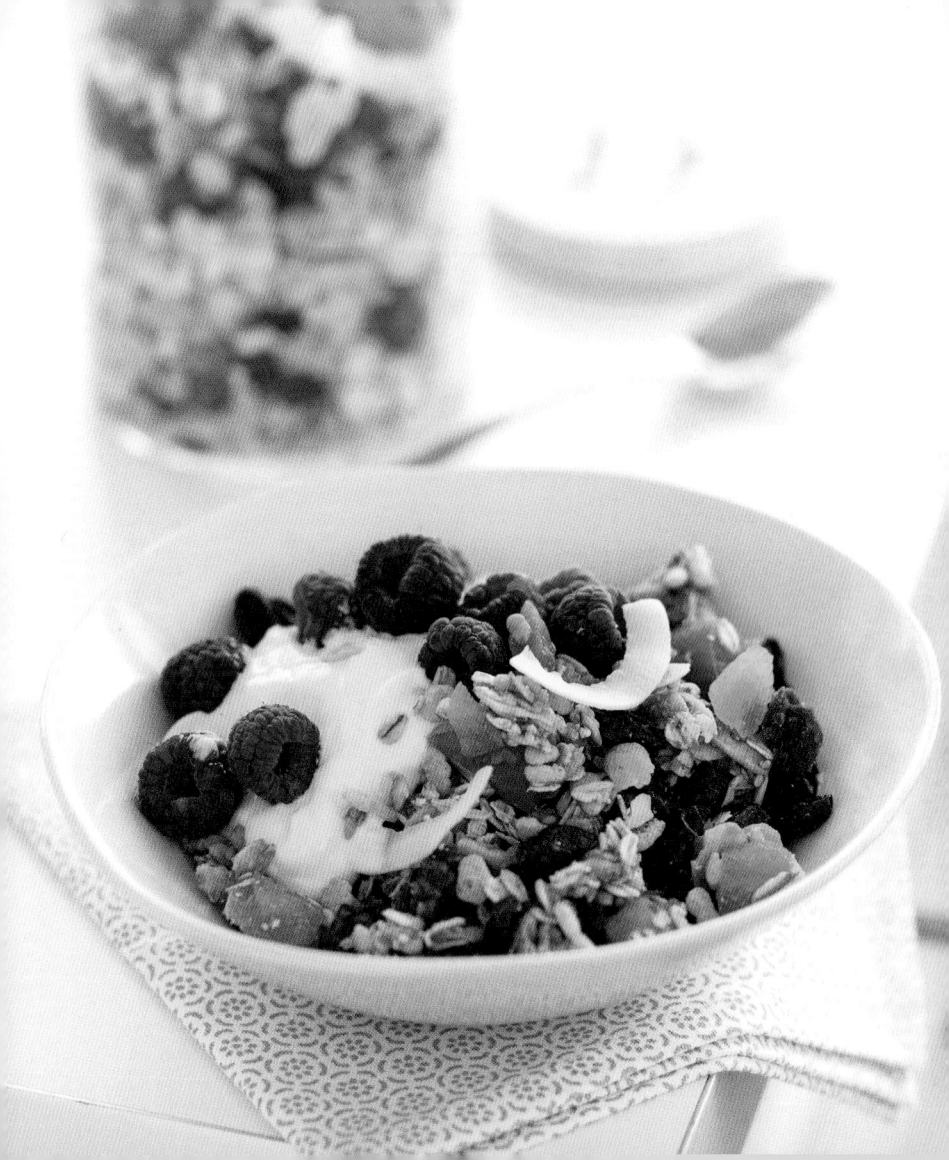

Classic apple pie

This pie is perfect after Sunday lunch all year round. Try adding a handful of blackberries in autumn, cranberries in winter, and some chopped rhubarb in spring.

TAKES 2¼–2½ HOURS ● SERVES 8

1kg/2lb 4oz Bramley apples, peeled, cored and thinly sliced
140g/5oz golden caster sugar, plus extra for sprinkling
½ tsp ground cinnamon
3 tbsp gluten-free plain flour
1 egg white, beaten with a fork
cream or ice cream, to serve

FOR THE PASTRY

225g/8oz cold butter, diced
400g/14oz gluten-free plain flour, plus a little extra for dusting
3 tbsp icing sugar
2 tsp xanthan gum
1 egg, beaten

1 To make the pastry, rub the butter into the flour until the mixture resembles fine breadcrumbs. Stir in the icing sugar and xanthan gum. Mix the egg with 4 tablespoons water, then mix into the dry ingredients with a cutlery knife until the dough starts to come together (add a tablespoon more water if you need to). Knead lightly, wrap in cling film and chill for 30 minutes.

2 Heat oven to 190C/170C fan/gas 5. Roll out two-thirds of the pastry to line a pie tin – 20–22cm round and 4cm deep – leaving a slight overhang.

3 Roll the remaining third to a circle about 28cm/11in in diameter. Mix the apples with the sugar and cinnamon. Pile into the tin.

4 Brush a little water around the pastry rim and lay the pastry lid over, pressing the edges together to seal. Trim the edge with a knife and poke a hole in the lid. Brush all over with egg white and sprinkle with sugar. Bake for 40–45 minutes, then remove and sit for 5–10 minutes.

PER SERVING 695 kcals, protein 9g, carbs 95g, fat 33g, sat fat 20g, fibre 4g, sugar 32g, salt 0.79g

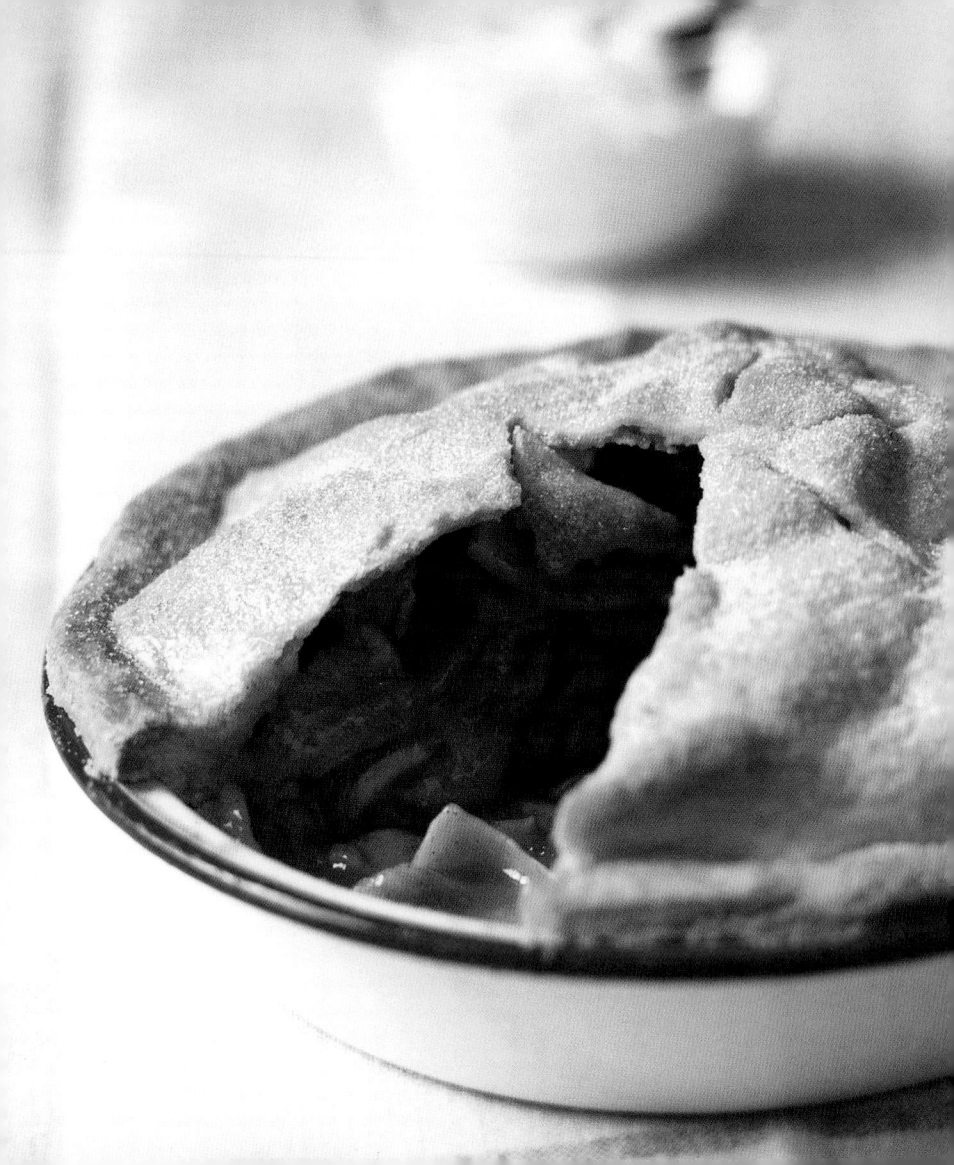

Hot cross buns

Happy Easter to you! These buns are best eaten on the day they are made, but leftovers will still be delicious toasted and spread with butter.

TAKES 1 HOUR • MAKES 15

300ml/½ pint warm full-fat milk, plus
   2 tbsp more
50g/2oz butter, melted
1 egg, beaten
500g/1lb 2oz gluten-free and
   wheat-free white bread flour
75g/2½oz caster sugar
2 tsp fast-action yeast
1 tbsp sunflower oil for greasing
75g/2½oz sultanas
50g/2oz mixed peel
zest 1 orange
1 tsp ground cinnamon
1 tsp sunflower oil, plus extra for
   shaping
3 tbsp apricot jam, melted and sieved

FOR THE CROSSES

75g/2½oz gluten-free plain flour

1 Whisk the milk, butter and egg together. Put the flour, 1 teaspoon of salt, sugar and yeast into a bowl. Make a well in the centre and pour in the milk mixture. Mix with a wooden spoon, then bring together with your hands to a sticky dough.

2 Put the dough in a lightly oiled bowl. Cover with oiled cling film and leave to rise in a warm place for 1 hour or until doubled in size.

3 Mix in the sultanas, peel, orange zest, cinnamon and oil. Leave to rise for 1 hour more, or until doubled in size, again covered by some well-oiled cling film.

4 Heat oven to 220C/200C fan/gas 7. Divide the dough into 100g/4oz pieces, lightly oil your hands and shape into buns. Sit on a baking sheet. For the crosses, mix the flour with about 5 tablespoons water to make a thick paste. Pipe a cross on each bun. Bake for 20 minutes on the middle shelf of the oven, until golden.

5 Brush warm apricot jam over the top of the warm buns.

PER BUN 226 kcals, protein 5g, carbs 41g, fat 4g, sat fat 2g, fibre 2g, sugar 14g, salt 0.5g

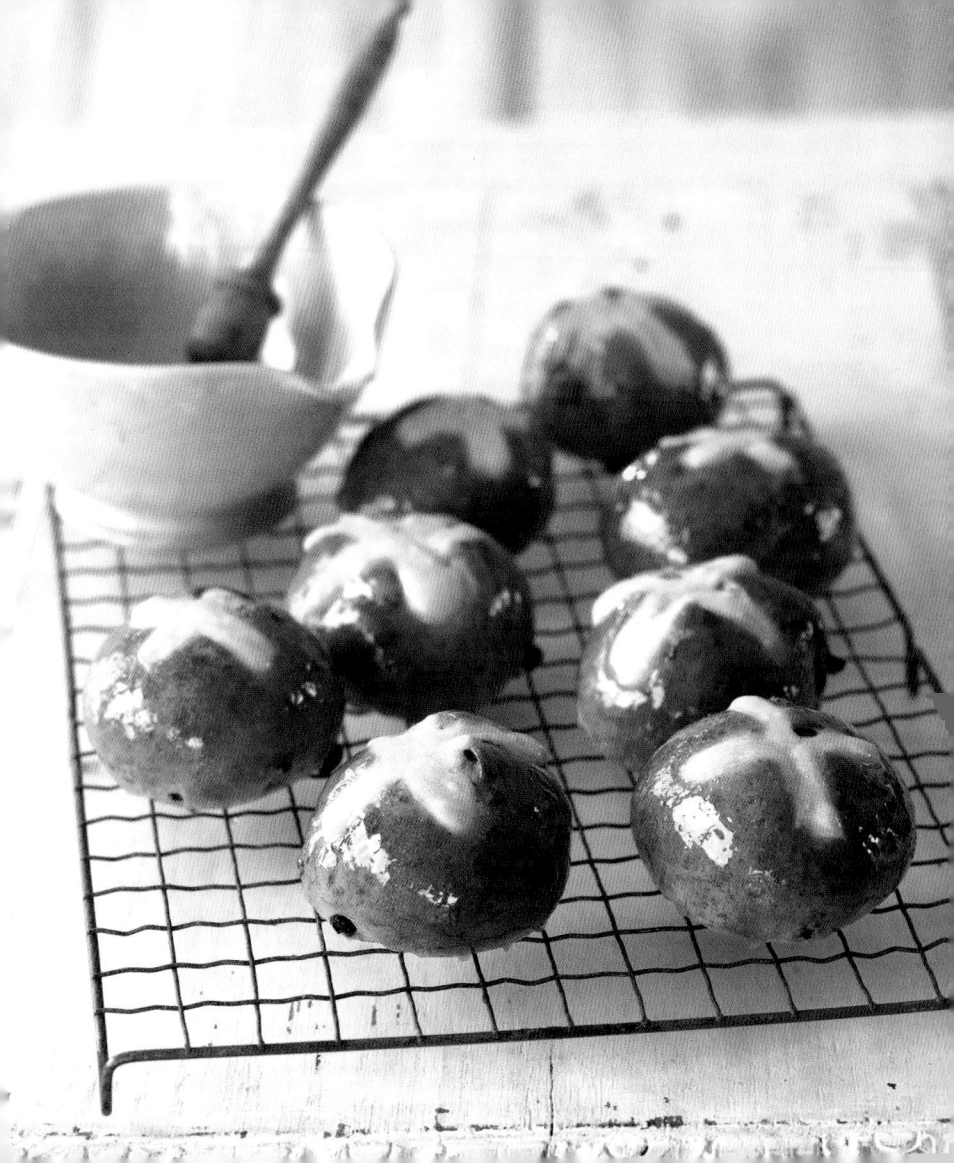

Lemon tart

Delicious served just as it is, or for a smarter occasion add single cream or crème fraîche to serve, plus a small handful of mixed berries.

TAKES 1½ HOURS, PLUS CHILLING
● **SERVES 8**
FOR THE PASTRY
300g/10oz gluten-free flour, plus extra
  for rolling
2 tbsp icing sugar
1 tsp xanthan gum
zest 1 lemon
140g/5oz butter, diced
1 egg, beaten
FOR THE FILLING
5 large eggs
140g/5oz caster sugar
150ml/¼ pint double cream
juice 2–3 lemons (about 100ml/3½fl oz)
2 tbsp lemon zest

1 Put the flour, icing sugar, gum, lemon zest, butter and ½ teaspoon salt into a food processor and whizz to fine crumbs. Mix the egg with 2 tablespoons water, then dribble into the food processor while whizzing, until the pastry starts to come together into a dough. Add 1 tablespoon more water at a time, if it needs it. Knead the dough for a few minutes, then wrap in cling film and chill for 30 minutes.
2 Beat all the filling ingredients, except for the zest, together. Sieve, then stir in the zest.
3 Roll out the pastry on a lightly floured surface to line a 23cm tart tin.
4 Heat oven to 200C/180C fan/gas 6. Line the tart with greaseproof paper and fill with baking beans. Bake for 15 minutes, then remove the paper and beans, and bake for another 15 minutes until biscuity. Pour in the lemon mixture and bake again for 30–35 minutes until just set. Leave to cool, then remove the tart from the tin and serve at room temperature or chilled.

PER SERVING 770 kcals, protein 13g, carbs 86g, fat 44g, sat fat 24g, fibre 2g, sugar 38g, salt 0.18g

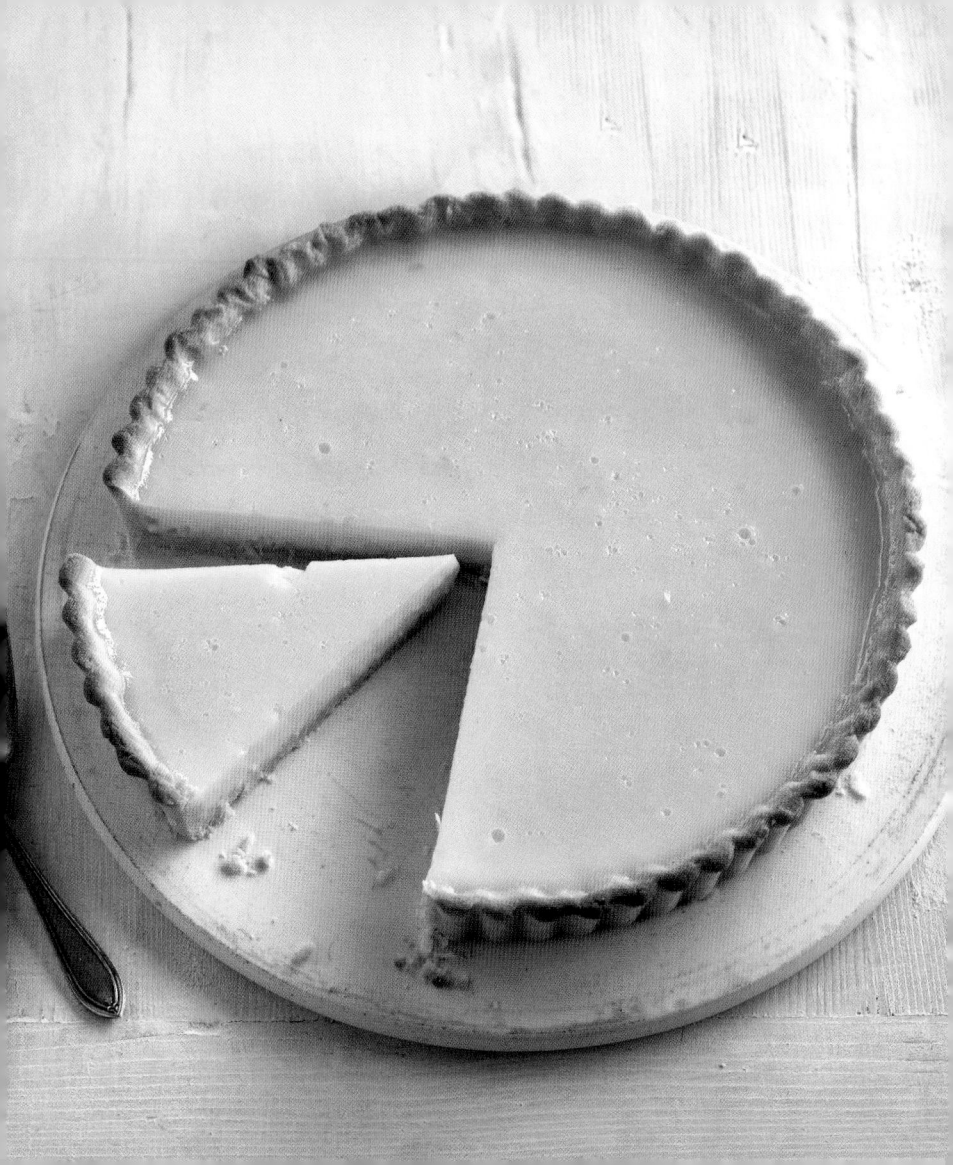

Pancakes

This is the basic recipe for crêpes and pancakes – you could add a pinch of ground cinnamon or even finely chopped herbs.

TAKES 30 MINUTES, PLUS RESTING
● **MAKES 12**

140g/5oz gluten-free plain flour
200ml/7fl oz whole milk
2 eggs
25g/1oz unsalted butter, melted, plus
  a little extra for greasing

1 Sift the flour with a pinch of salt into a bowl and make a well in the middle. Mix the milk and 100ml/3½fl oz water together. Break the eggs into the well and start whisking slowly. Add the milk and water in a steady stream, whisking constantly and gradually incorporating the flour.

2 Whisk until the batter is smooth and all the flour has been incorporated. Set aside for 30 minutes, then whisk in the butter.

3 Heat the pan over a medium heat. Lightly grease the pan with melted butter. Using a ladle, pour about 2 tablespoons of batter into the pan and swirl it around so the bottom of the pan is evenly coated. You want to use just enough batter to make a delicate, lacy pancake. Cook the pancake for about 45 seconds on one side until golden and then flip the pancake over and cook the other side for about 30 seconds until it freckles.

4 Slide the pancake out of the pan and either serve immediately or stack on a plate with baking parchment in between.

PER PANCAKE 84 kcals, protein 3g, carbs 10g, fat 4g, sat fat 2g, fibre none, sugar 1g, salt 0.06g

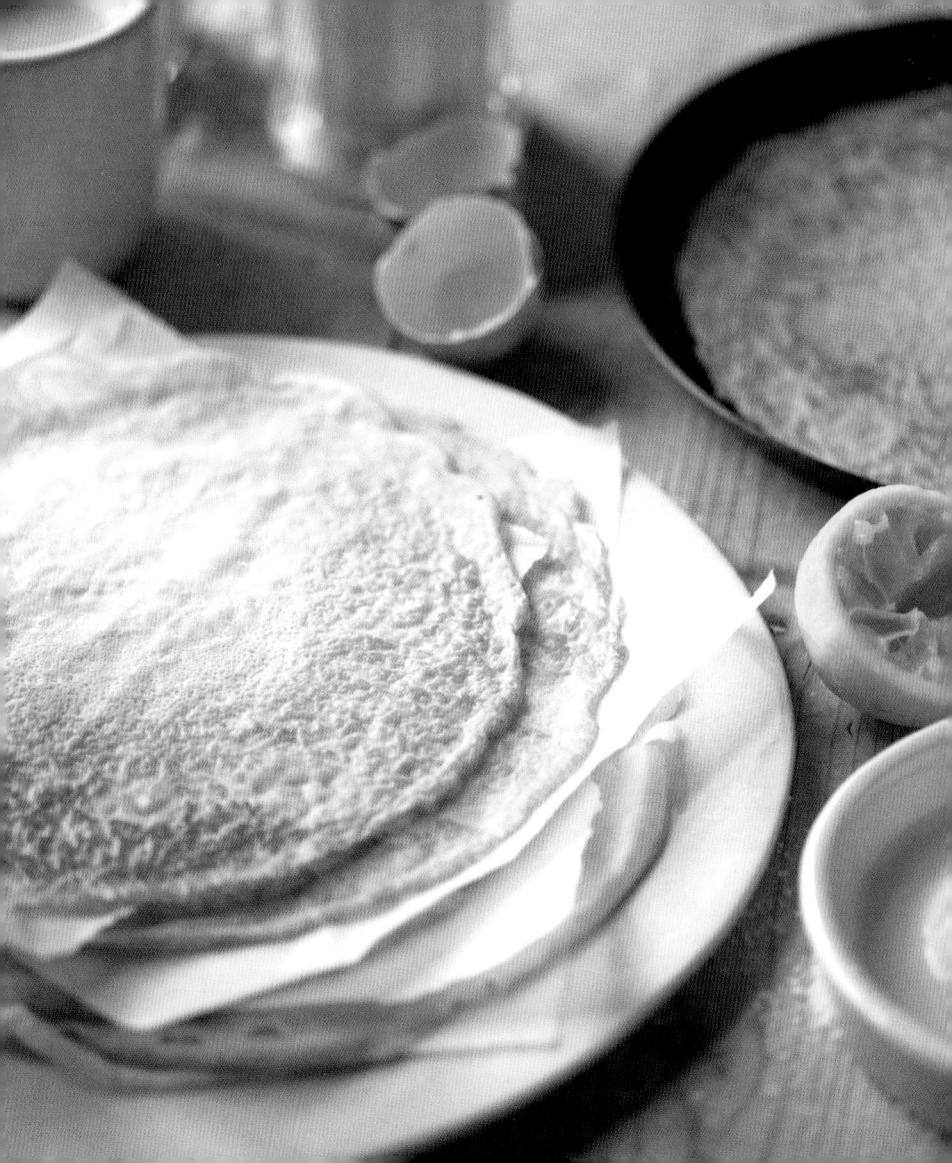

Raspberry bakewell

This is perfect as a warm pud with custard, or leave to cool and eat slices with a cup of tea.

TAKES 1 HOUR 20 MINUTES, PLUS CHILLING • SERVES 10

5 tbsp seedless raspberry jam
100g/4oz raspberries
25g/1oz flaked almonds
4 tbsp apricot jam

FOR THE PASTRY

175g/5oz cold butter, diced, plus extra
    for greasing
300g/10oz gluten-free plain flour, plus
    a little extra for dusting
1½ tsp xanthan gum
1½ tbsp icing sugar

FOR THE SPONGE

200g/7oz butter, very soft
200g/7oz golden caster sugar
100g/4oz ground almonds
100g/4oz gluten-free plain flour
2 tsp gluten-free baking powder
½ tsp almond extract
4 eggs, beaten

1 To make the pastry, rub the butter into the flour to fine breadcrumbs. Stir in the xanthan gum and icing sugar. Add 6 tablespoons water, mixing with a cutlery knife until the dough starts to come together. Knead lightly, roll into a log, wrap in cling film and chill for 30 minutes.

2 Heat oven to 200C/180C fan/gas 6. Line the base and sides of a buttered 20 × 30 cm traybake tin, with parchment. Slice the pastry into disks the thickness of a £1 coin and press into the tin to line with no gaps. Prick with a fork; chill for 20 minutes.

3 Bake the pastry for 15 minutes until just cooked. Cool for a few minutes and turn down the oven to 180C/160C fan/gas 4. Dot the raspberry jam over the pastry and scatter over the raspberries.

4 For the sponge, beat all the ingredients with an electric whisk until smooth. Spoon over the raspberry layer, then smooth evenly. Scatter over the flaked almonds and bake for 35–40 minutes. Brush apricot jam over the top just before serving.

PER SERVING 652 kcals, protein 7.5g, carbs 64g, fat 40g, sat fat 21g, fibre 1.1g, sugar 32g, salt 1g

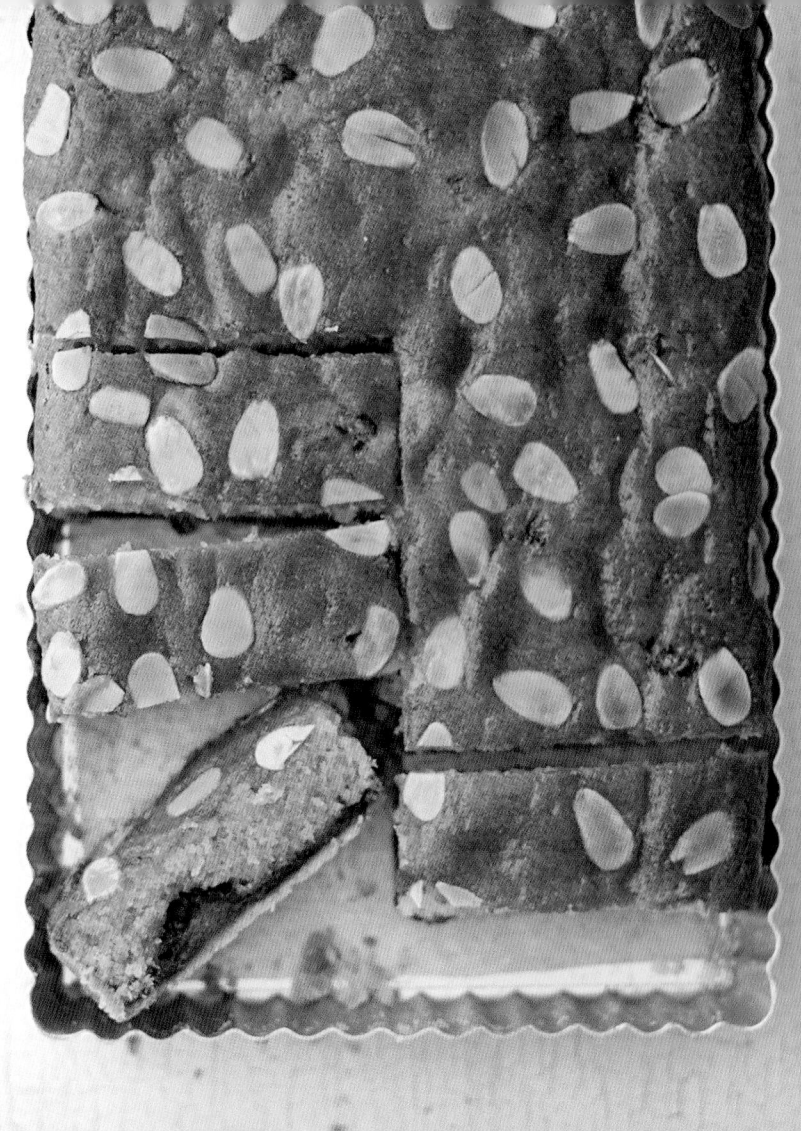

Schooldays treacle sponge

This nostalgic recipe will take you back. Save it until the weather is cold and miserable, and cheer yourself up with this comfort food classic.

TAKES 2 HOURS • SERVES 4 GENEROUSLY

175g/6oz unsalted butter, softened, plus extra for greasing

3 tbsp golden syrup, plus extra for drizzling (optional)

1 tbsp gluten-free white breadcrumbs

175g/6oz golden caster sugar

zest 1 lemon

3 large eggs, beaten

175g/6oz gluten-free plain flour

1 tsp gluten-free baking powder

2 tbsp milk

custard or clotted cream, to serve

1 Use a small knob of butter to heavily grease a 2-litre pudding basin. In a small bowl, mix the golden syrup with the breadcrumbs then tip into the pudding basin.

2 Beat the butter with the sugar and zest until light and fluffy, then add the eggs gradually. Fold in the flour, then the baking powder, then finally add the milk.

3 Spoon the mix into the pudding basin. Cover with a double layer of buttered foil and baking paper, making a pleat in the centre to allow the pudding to rise. Tie the foil securely with string, then put in a steamer or large pan containing enough gently simmering water to come halfway up the sides of the basin. Steam for 1½ hours. Turn out on to a serving dish. Serve drizzled with extra golden syrup, if you like, and lashings of custard or clotted cream.

PER SERVING 763 kcals, protein 10g, carbs 90g, fat 43g, sat fat 25g, fibre 1g, sugar 56g, salt 0.71g

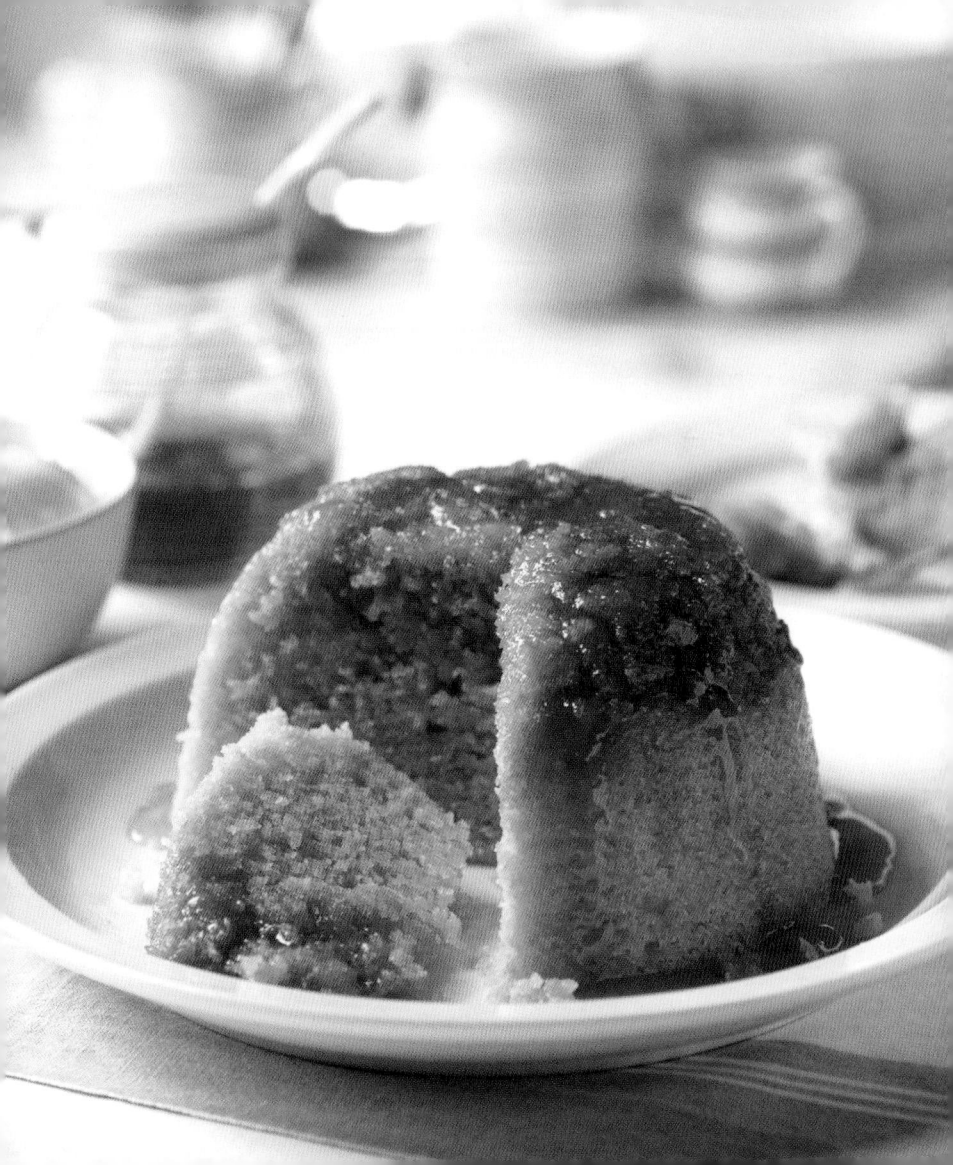

English scones

Best eaten freshly baked with lots of berry jam, clotted cream and a pot of tea.

TAKES 30 MINUTES ● MAKES 10–12

450g/1lb gluten-free self-raising flour
(check the ingredients, add 1 tsp
xanthan gum if it doesn't contain
any), plus extra for dusting
1 tsp bicarbonate of soda
100g/4oz cold butter, diced
85g/3oz golden caster sugar
284ml pot buttermilk
2 tsp vanilla extract
splash milk

1 Heat oven to 220C/200C fan/gas 7. Put the flour, bicarb, ¼ teaspoon salt and butter into a food processor and pulse until you can't feel any lumps of butter (or rub in the butter with your fingers). Pulse in the sugar.

2 Gently warm the buttermilk (don't throw away the pot) and vanilla in a microwave or pan. Using your largest bowl, quickly tip in some of the flour mix, followed by some of the buttermilk mix, repeating until everything is in the bowl. Use a knife to quickly mix together to form a dough – don't overmix it.

3 Tip on to a floured surface and lightly bring together with your hands a couple of times. Press out gently to about 4cm/1½in thick and stamp out rounds with a 6cm or 7cm cutter. Re-shape the trimmings until all the dough is used.

4 Spread the scones out on a lightly floured baking sheet or two. Add a splash of milk into the buttermilk pot, then use to glaze the top of each scone. Bake for 10–12 minutes until golden and well risen.

PER SCONE (12) 229 kcals, protein 4g, carbs 39g, fat 8g, sat fat 5g, fibre 1g, sugar 10g, salt 0.6g

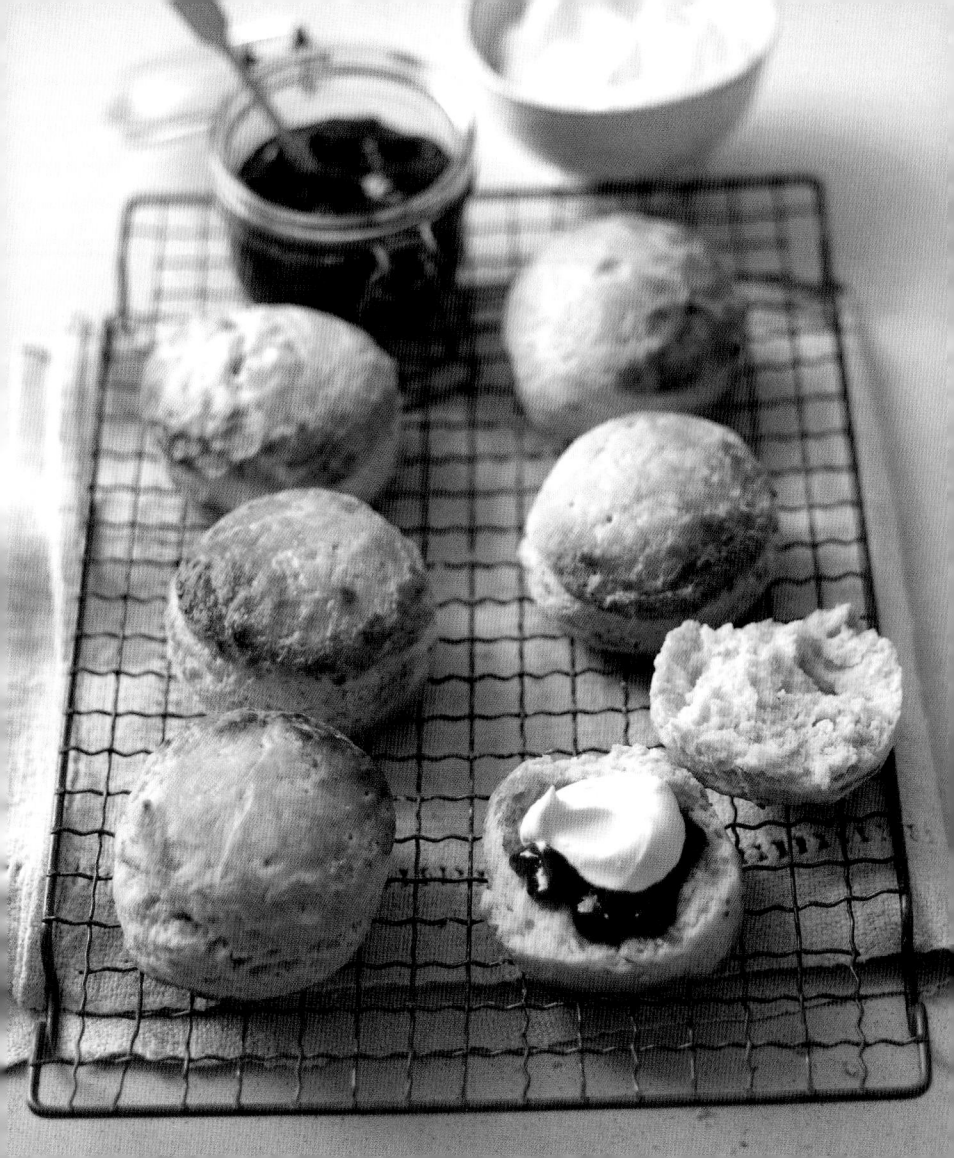

Apple & blackberry crumble

A simple yet richly comforting dessert. By pre-cooking the crumble mixture you avoid an uncooked, gluey topping and retain the texture of the fruit.

TAKES 40 MINUTES ● SERVES 4

FOR THE CRUMBLE TOPPING
120g/4½oz gluten-free plain flour
25g/1oz ground almonds
5 tbsp caster sugar
85g/3oz cold butter, cut into pieces

FOR THE FRUIT
300g/10oz eating apples
2 tbsp demerara sugar
120g/4½oz blackberries
¼ tsp ground cinnamon
custard or vanilla ice cream, to serve

1 Heat oven to 190C/170C fan/gas 5. Tip the flour, almonds and sugar into a large bowl. Add the butter, then rub into the flour using your fingertips until the mixture resembles breadcrumbs. Do not overwork it or the crumble will become heavy. Sprinkle the mixture evenly over a baking sheet and bake for 15 minutes or until lightly coloured.

2 Meanwhile, for the fruit, peel, core and cut the apples into 2cm/¾in dice. Put the apples and sugar in a medium pan and cook for 5 minutes until almost softened. Add the blackberries and cinnamon, and cook for 3–4 minutes more.

3 To serve, spoon the fruit into an ovenproof dish, top with the crumble mix, then bake in the oven for 10–15 minutes until hot through. Serve with hot custard or vanilla ice cream.

PER SERVING 395 kcals, protein 4g, carbs 56g, fat 19g, sat fat 12g, fibre 3g, sugar 33g, salt 0.02g

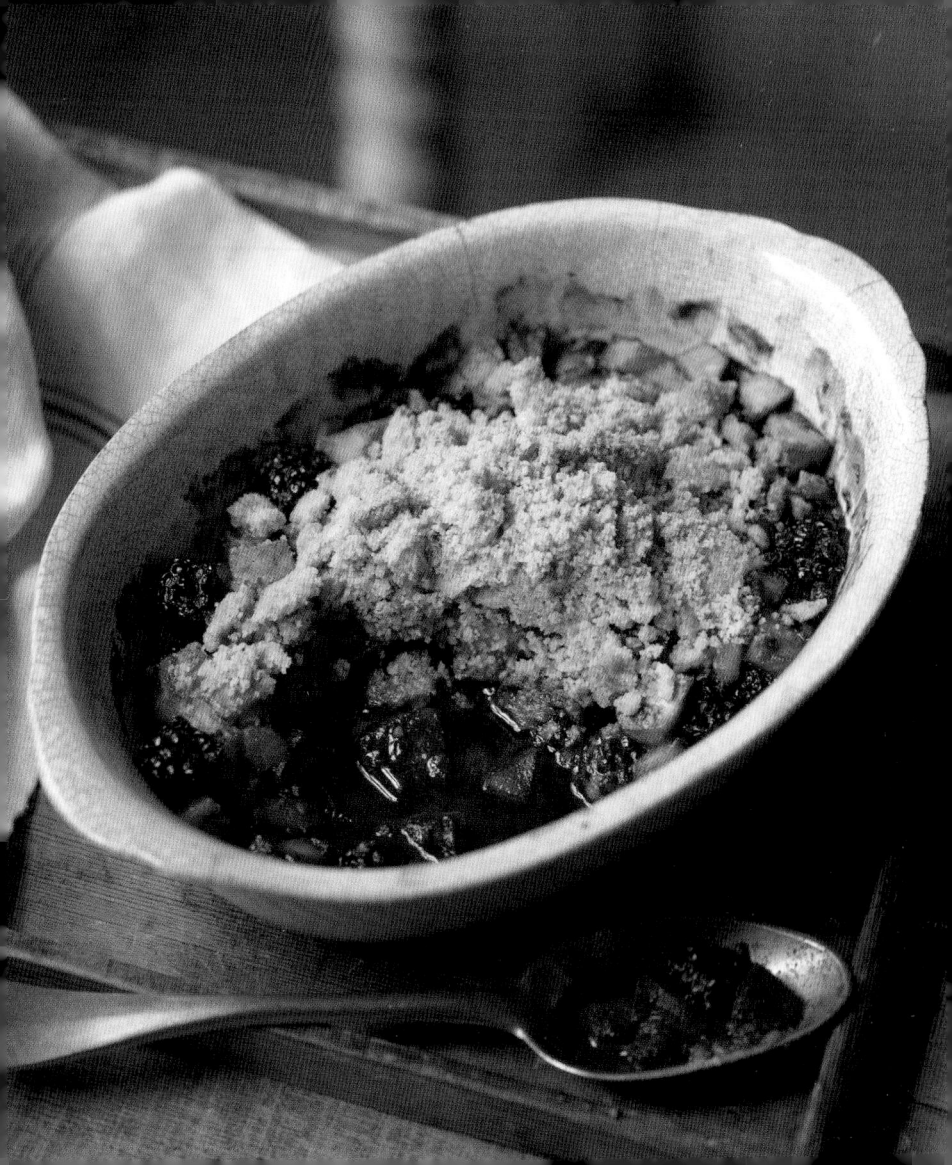

Mince pies

Choose your favourite topping, or make a few of each. These pies can all be frozen, uncooked and wrapped in cling film, for up to a month before baking.

TAKES 45 MINUTES, PLUS CHILLING

● **MAKES 12**

120g/4½oz cold butter, diced
200g/7oz gluten-free plain flour, plus a little extra for dusting
1 tbsp icing sugar
about 300g/10oz gluten-free mincemeat

FOR THE FESTIVE STAR TOPS

pastry trimmings
2 tbsp granulated sugar

FOR THE CRUMBLE TOPPING

50g/2oz cold butter, diced
7 tbsp gluten-free plain flour
5 tbsp demerara sugar
1½ tsp ground cinnamon

FOR THE CRUNCHY ALMOND TOPPING

100g/4oz gluten-free marzipan, coarsely grated
50g/2oz toasted flaked almonds

1 To make the pastry, follow the instructions on p148.

2 Heat oven to 180C/160C fan/gas 4. On a lightly floured surface, roll the pastry out to a 2–3mm thickness. Using an 8cm cutter, stamp out 12 discs, re-rolling the trimmings, if you need to. Line a bun tin with the pastry discs, then spoon a little mincemeat into each.

3 For the festive star tops, roll out the remaining pastry and pat on sugar. Use a small star cutter to stamp out 12 shapes and add one to each. For the crumble, rub together the butter, flour, sugar and cinnamon. Sprinkle over the pies. Or for a crunchy almond topping, mix the marzipan and almonds, and scatter over.

4 Bake on the middle shelf of the oven for about 20 minutes until the pastry is cooked and golden brown.

PER FESTIVE STAR PIE 245 kcals, protein 1.8g, carbs 37g, fat 11g, sat fat 4g, fibre 1g, sugar 24g, salt 0.17g: PER CRUMBLE PIE 311 kcals, protein 2g, carbs 46g, fat 15g, sat fat 6g, fibre 1g, sugar 28g, salt 0.22g: PER CRUNCHY MARZIPAN PIE 294 kcals, protein 3g, carbs 41g, fat 14g, sat fat 4g, fibre 2g, sugar 28g, salt 0.18g

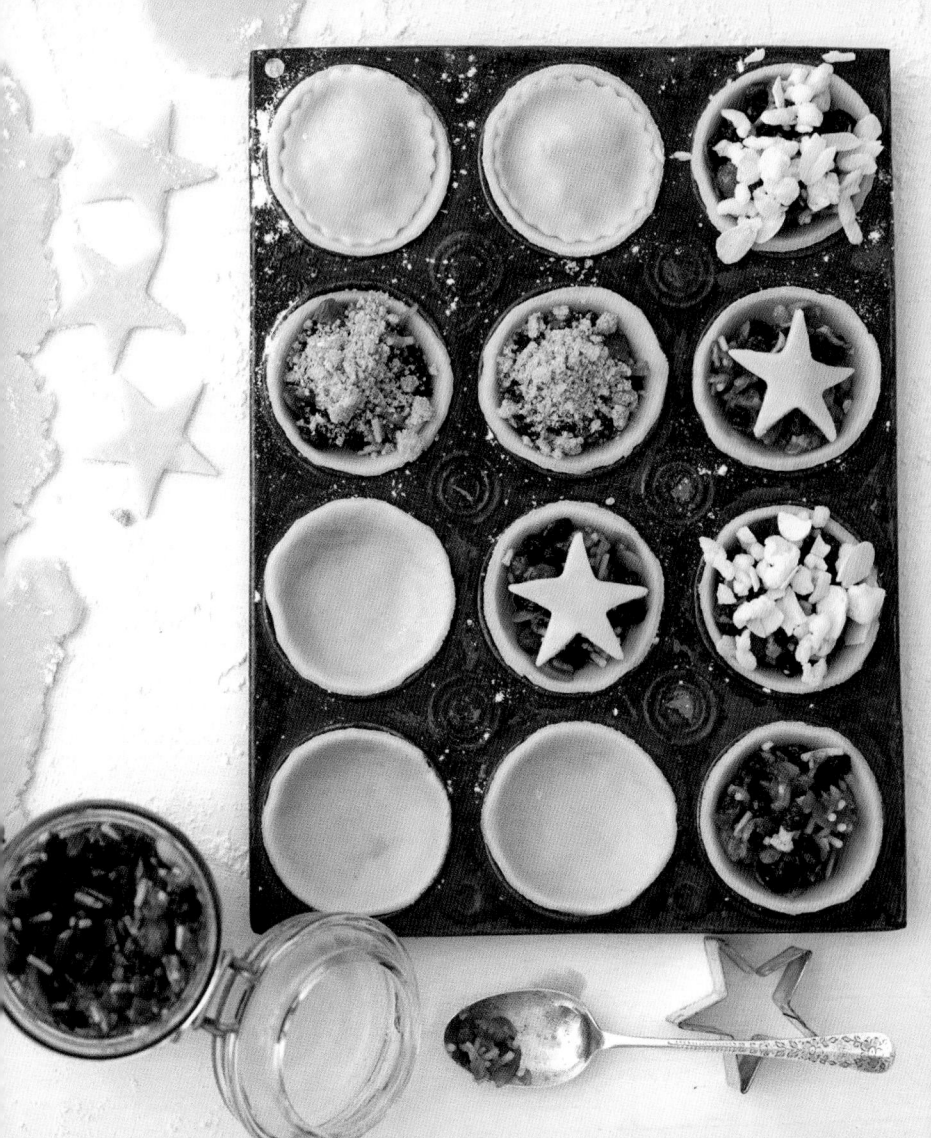

Snowy Christmas cakes

This square cake is cut into two loaf-shaped cakes, so you give one to a friend, or keep one spare for when guests call round.

TAKES 3 HOURS, PLUS SOAKING OVERNIGHT • MAKES 2 CAKES

550g/1lb 4oz mixed dried fruit
150ml/¼ pint sherry
zest and juice 2 clementines or satsumas
140g/5oz gluten-free plain flour
1 tsp each xanthan gum and gluten-free baking powder
2 tsp ground mixed spice
140g/5oz unsalted butter, softened, plus extra for greasing
140g/5oz soft dark brown sugar
3 medium eggs
50g/2oz ground almonds
100g/4oz glacé cherries, washed and halved
50g/2oz pecan nuts, chopped

TO DECORATE

250g pack gluten-free marzipan, halved
icing sugar, for dusting
2 tbsp warmed apricot jam
500g pack fondant icing sugar
8 glacé cherries and small holly sprigs, washed and dried

1 Heat the dried fruit, sherry, clementine or satsuma zest and juice in a pan, then cover and leave overnight.

2 Heat oven to 150C/130C fan/gas 2. Grease and line the base and sides of a deep, square 18cm cake tin with baking parchment. Mix the flour, xanthan gum, baking powder and spice.

3 In a big bowl, beat the butter, sugar, eggs, flour, xantham gum, baking powder, spice and almonds. Stir in the soaked fruit and juices, cherries and pecans.

4 Spoon into the tin and bake for 1½–2 hours or until a skewer inserted comes out clean. Cool in the tin.

5 Cut the cake in half and trim the edges. Roll out each piece of marzipan on a surface dusted with icing sugar. Brush the cake tops with jam, put jam-side down on the marzipan and trim the excess.

6 Make up the fondant icing to a spreading consistency, then spread on top of the cakes. Top with cherries and holly, then leave to set. Keeps for a week.

PER SERVING 479 kcals, protein 5g, carbs 81g, fat 14g, sat fat 5g, fibre 1.7g, sugar 75g, salt 0.2g

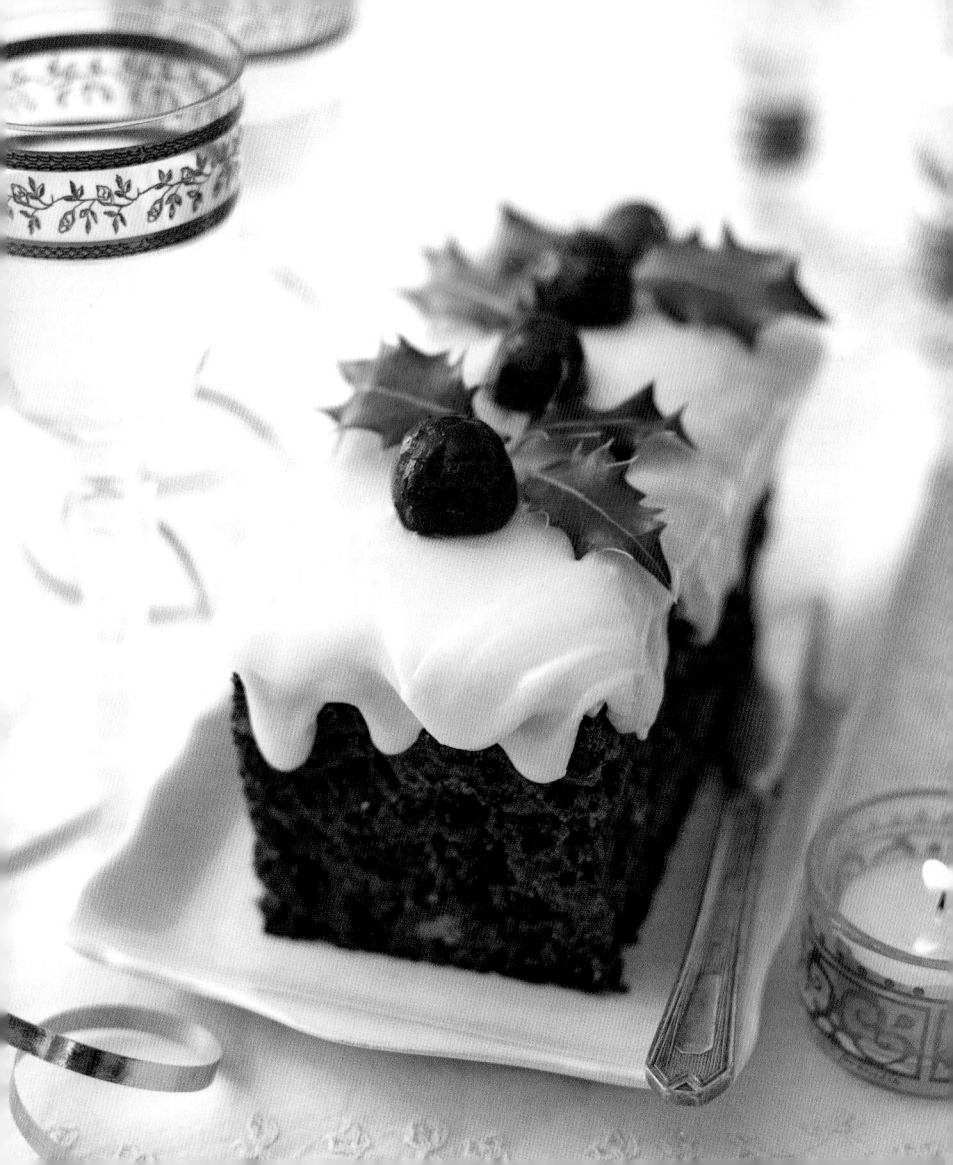

Christmas pudding

Christmas just wouldn't be Christmas without a traditional pud for the whole family to share. Just add custard, brandy butter and cream for the full works.

TAKES 5 HOURS, PLUS COOLING
● **SERVES 8**

500g/1lb 2oz mixed dried fruit
50g/2oz dried cranberries
4 tbsp brandy
125ml/4fl oz gluten-free dark beer
120g/4½oz unsalted butter, softened
225g/8oz dark soft brown sugar
2 eggs, beaten
1 tsp mixed spice
½ tsp ground cinnamon
grating fresh nutmeg
100g/4oz ground almonds
1 tsp gluten-free baking powder
grated zest 1 orange
grated zest 1 lemon
1 Bramley apple, peeled and grated

1 Tip the dried fruit, brandy and beer into a medium-sized pan and heat gently for 2 minutes until the fruit has started to absorb the liquid. Cool.

2 In a bowl beat together the butter and sugar. Gradually add the eggs. In another bowl, combine the spices, ground almonds and baking powder. Add to the butter-mix with the grated zests and apple. Stir well, then stir in the dried fruit mixture.

3 Butter a 1.2-litre pudding basin and put a buttered disc of parchment in the bottom. Spoon in the mixture and cover with a pleated square of greaseproof paper and foil. Tie securely with string; cut off any excess paper and foil. Place in a pan and pour enough boiling water to come two-thirds of the way up the sides of the bowl. Cover the pan and cook at a gentle simmer for 4½ hours, topping up the water as necessary. Cool, then store in a cool, dry cupboard for up to a year.

4 To serve, re-boil the pud as above for 1–2 hours until hot through.

PER SERVING 581 kcals, protein 8g, carbs 81g, fat 25g, sat fat 10g, fibre 3g, sugar 78g, salt 0.37g

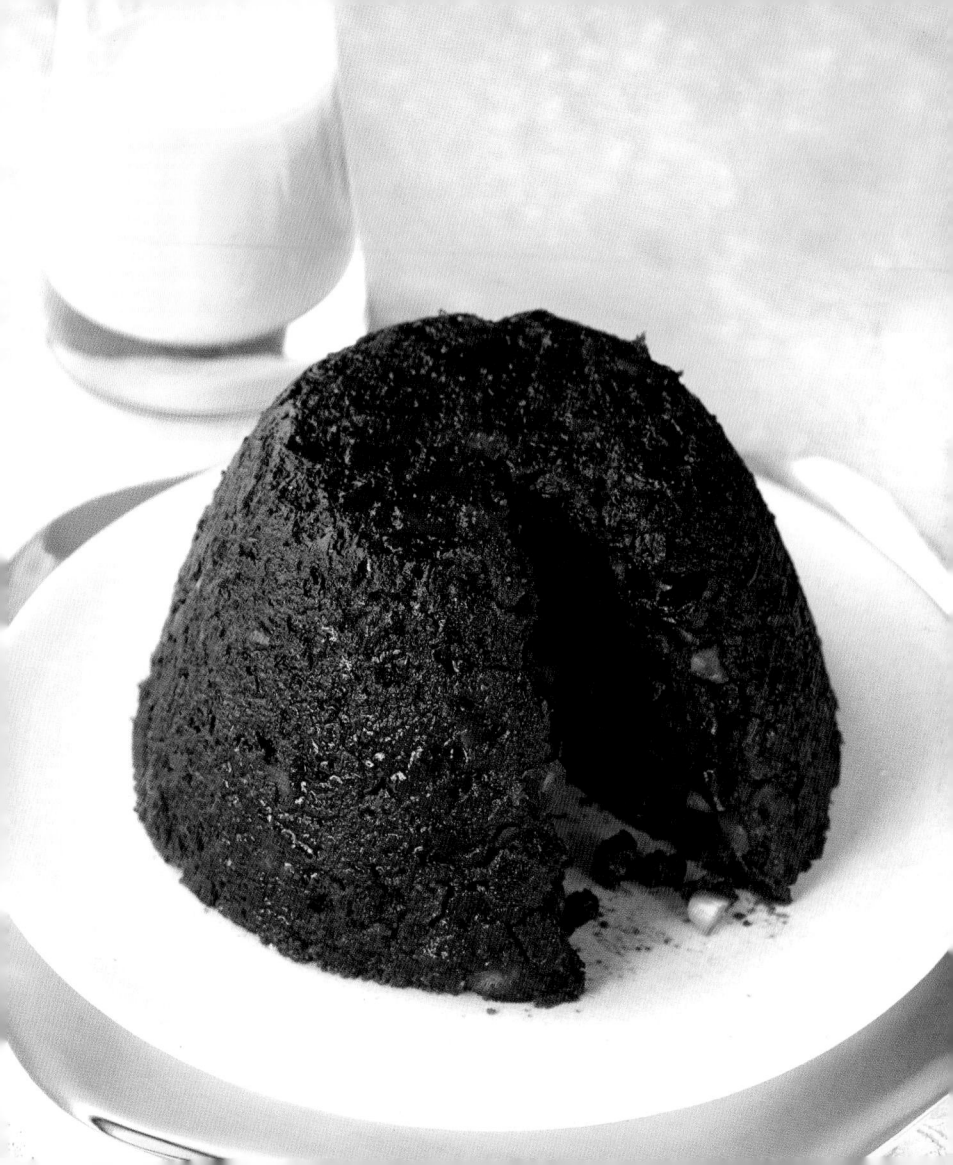

Right-every-time roasties

The secret to perfect roast potatoes is a good dusting of flour along with the oil, but polenta makes a great gluten-free alternative.

TAKES 1 HOUR 10 MINUTES

● **SERVES 8**

2kg/4lb 8oz roasting potatoes, such as King Edward, peeled

1 tbsp gluten-free plain flour

2 tbsp polenta

5 tbsp goose fat

5 tbsp vegetable oil

1 Cut the potatoes into quarters, or eighths, if really large – you want to end up with even-sized 5cm/2in pieces. Put the potatoes in a large lidded pan of salted water and boil for 5 minutes, just until the outside of the potato starts to soften. Drain really well.

2 Return to the pan and scatter over the flour, polenta and a little salt. Put the lid on top of the pan and give it a couple of good shakes, coating the potatoes in the flour and polenta and lightly crushing the sides.

3 Heat oven to 190C/170C fan/gas 5. Put the goose fat and oil in a roasting tin large enough to hold all the potatoes in one layer and heat in the oven for 5 minutes. Quickly tip the potatoes in and return to the oven. Cook for 30 minutes, turning once, then increase the heat to 220C/200C fan/gas 7. Cook for 20 minutes more or until crisp all over. Sprinkle with a little more salt, then serve.

PER SERVING 345 kcals, protein 6g, carbs 46g, fat 17g, sat fat 4g, fibre 3g, sugar 2g, salt 0.67g

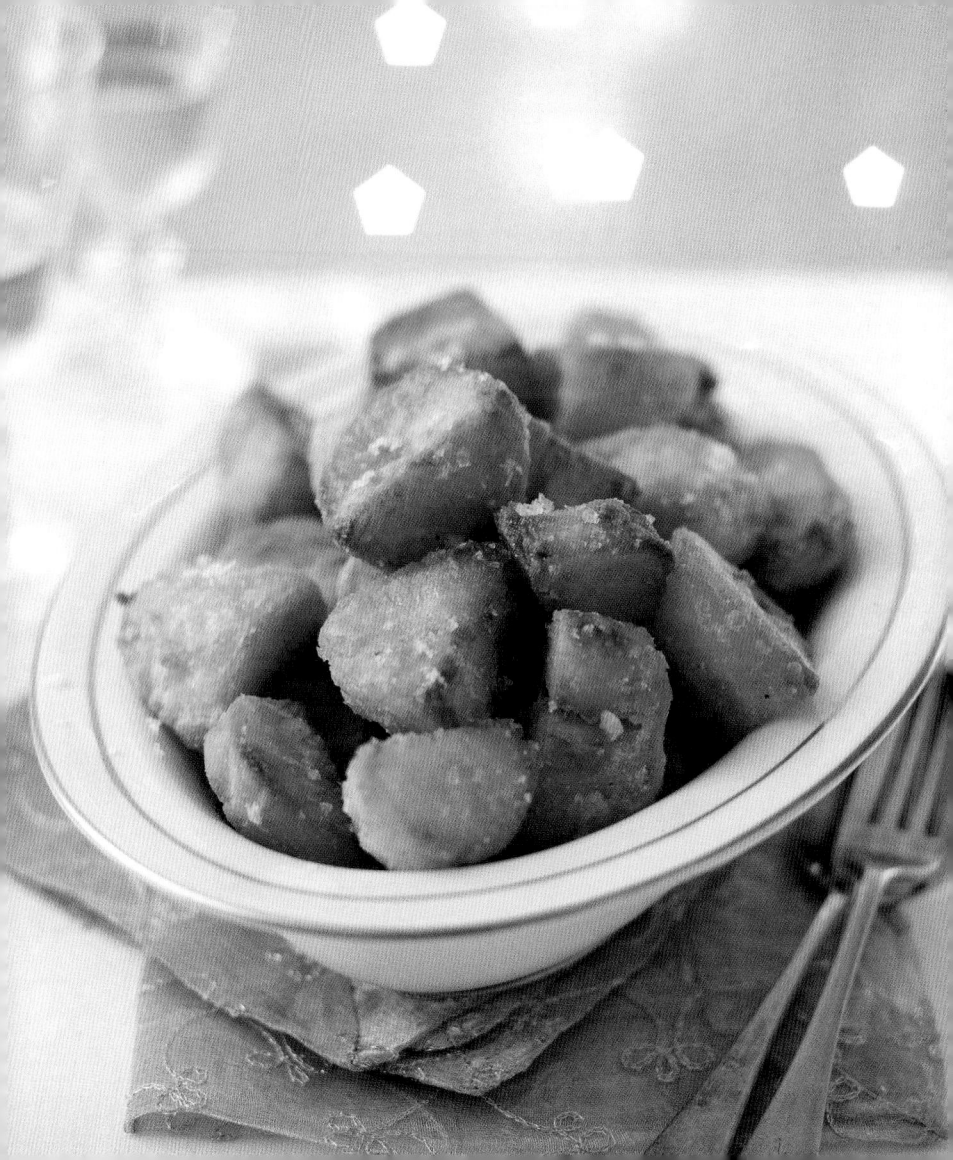

Yorkshire puddings

The secret to gloriously puffed-up Yorkshires is to have the fat sizzling hot – and don't open the oven door!

TAKES 30 MINUTES • MAKES 8 LARGE OR 24 SMALL

140g/5oz gluten-free plain flour
50g/2oz cornflour
3 eggs
175ml/6fl oz semi-skimmed milk
sunflower oil, for drizzling

1 Make up the batter mix. Tip the flours into a bowl with ½ teaspoon salt, make a well in the middle and crack the eggs into it. Whisk it together, then slowly add the milk, whisking all the time until lump-free. Leave to stand until you are ready to cook.

2 Heat oven to 230C/210C fan/gas 8. Drizzle a little oil evenly two 4-hole Yorkshire pudding tins or two 12-hole non-stick muffin tins and put in the oven to heat through.

3 Pour the batter into a jug, then remove the hot tins from the oven. Carefully and evenly pour the batter into the holes. Put the tins back in the oven and leave undisturbed for 20–25 minutes until the puddings have puffed up and browned. Serve immediately.

PER PUD (8 large) 199 kcals, protein 6g, carbs 15g, fat 13g, sat fat 2g, fibre none, sugar 1g, salt 0.12g

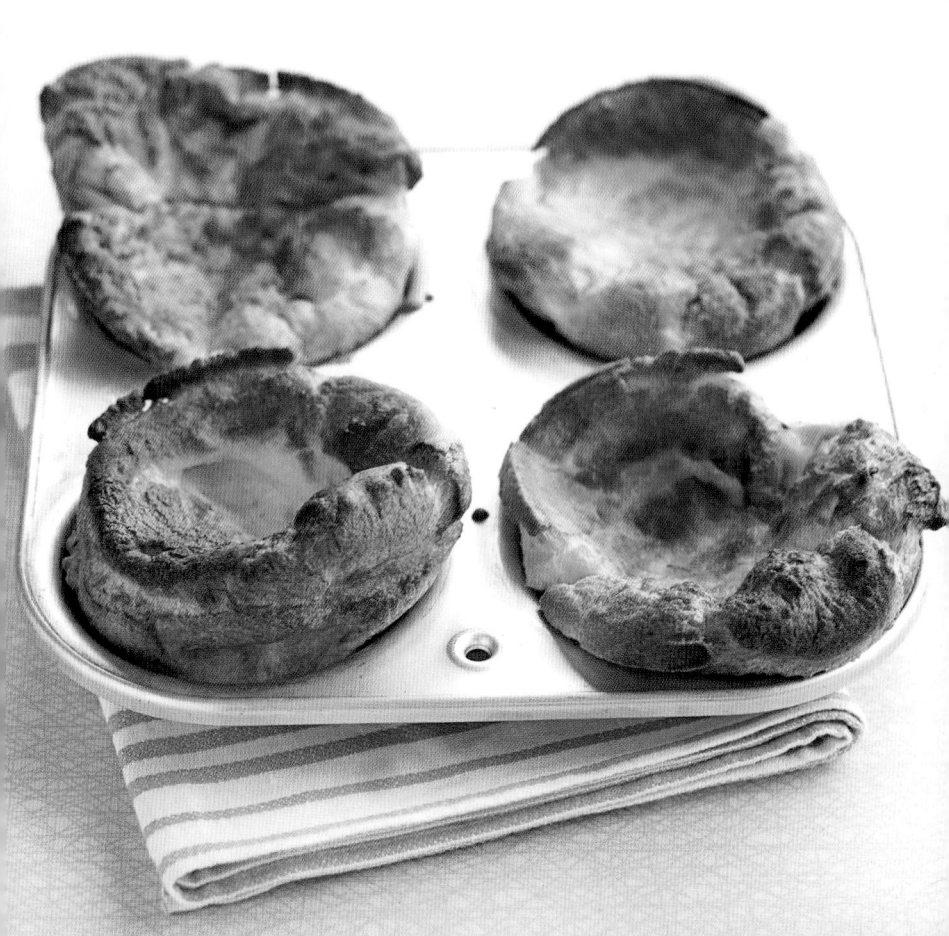

Homemade pizza

We've added ham, ricotta and pesto to these pizzas, but use whatever are your favourite toppings.

TAKES 1¼ HOURS ● SERVES 4

6–8 tbsp tomato pasta sauce

your favourite pizza toppings

FOR THE DOUGH

450g/1lb gluten-free plain flour, plus
 extra for dusting

2 tsp xanthan gum

2 tsp caster sugar

1 × 7g sachet fast-action dried yeast

2 eggs, beaten

6 tbsp olive oil, plus extra for greasing

1 For the dough, mix the flour, gum, sugar, yeast and 1 teaspoon salt in a bowl. Make a well in the centre and add the eggs, oil and 250ml/9fl oz hand-warm water, and stir in with a wooden spoon to a sticky dough. Knead for 5 minutes on a lightly floured surface then sit in an oiled bowl, cover with a clean tea towel and leave somewhere warm-ish to rise for 30 minutes.

2 Heat oven to 220C/200C fan/gas 7. Divide the dough into two and roll into pizza bases on a flour-dusted surface. Scatter a little flour on two baking sheets and lift on the pizza bases. Spread 3–4 tablespoons tomato sauce on each pizza base, then add your choice of toppings.

3 Bake for 20 minutes until the base is cooked through and crisp.

PER SERVING 282 kcals, protein 13g, carbs 43g, fat 7g, sat fat 3g, fibre 1g, sugar 4g, salt 1.51g

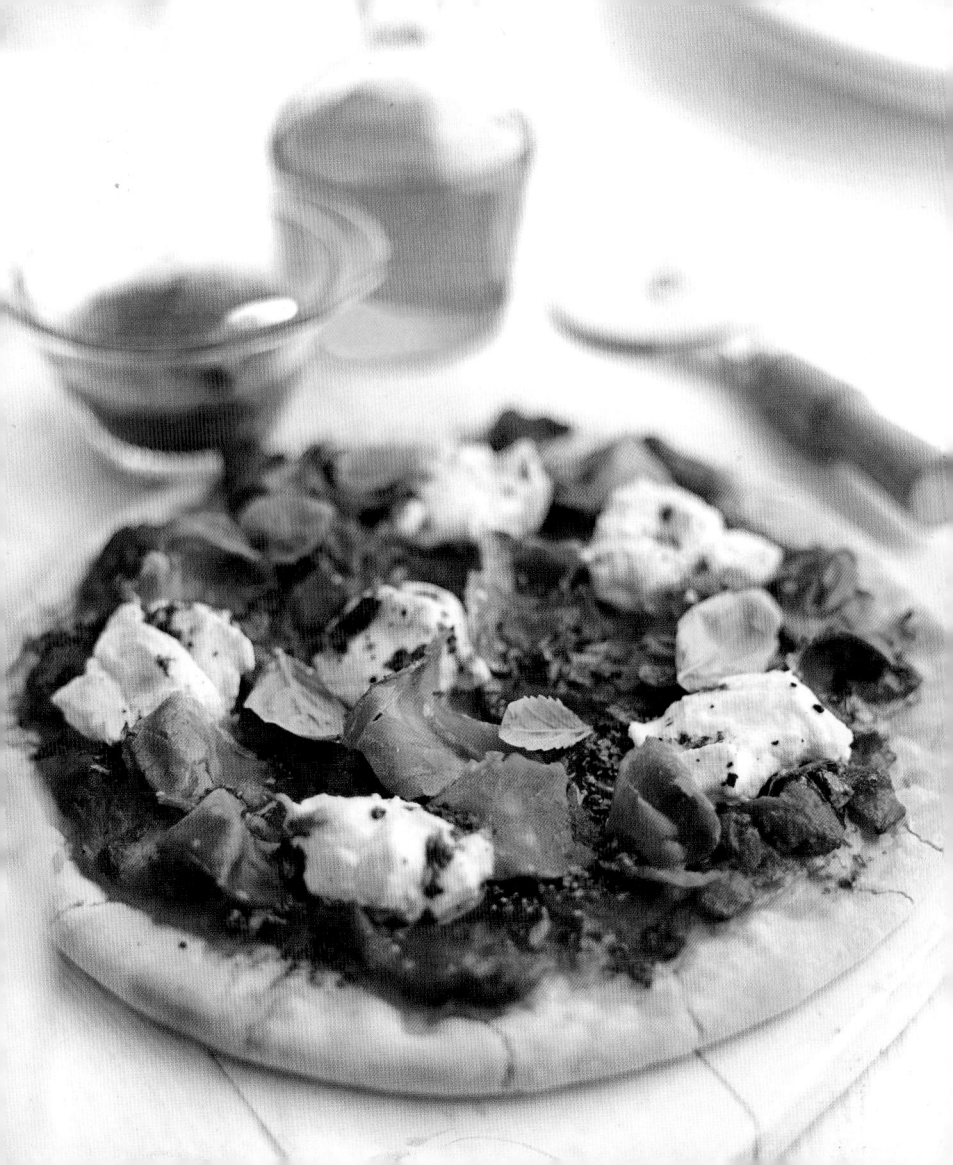

Lasagne

The lasagnes can be chilled in the fridge for 2 days before baking, or frozen for up to 3 months.

TAKES 3 HOURS • SERVES 10

3 tbsp olive oil
4 onions, finely chopped
8 garlic cloves, crushed
1 tbsp dried mixed herbs
2 bay leaves
1kg/2lb 4oz minced beef
4 × 400g cans chopped tomatoes
4 tbsp tomato purée
2 beef stock cubes, crumbled
small glass red wine (optional)
18–20 gluten-free no-cook lasagne
   sheets

FOR THE WHITE SAUCE

1.7 litres/3 pints milk
75g/2½oz cornflour
85g/3oz Parmesan, grated, plus extra
   to finish
few gratings nutmeg

1 For the meat sauce, heat the oil in a large pan and gently cook the onions for 10 minutes. Add the garlic, herbs, bay, beef, tomatoes, purée, stock cubes and wine, if using, or water. Bring to a simmer, breaking up the meat, and cook gently for 1 hour until saucy. Season.

2 Make the white sauce. In a large pan mix nine tablespoons of the milk to a paste with the cornflour. Gradually stir in the remaining milk. Bring to the boil, stirring, until thickened and smooth. Stir in the cheese with seasoning. If not using now, cover the surface with cling film.

3 Spread a thin layer of meat sauce into one or two baking dishes. Drizzle with a little white sauce and cover with a layer of lasagne sheets. Top with more of both sauces and more lasagne sheets. Repeat once more, then cover the top layer of lasagne in just white sauce. Scatter over some more Parmesan.

4 Heat oven to 200C/180C fan/ gas 6. Cook for 35–40 minutes.

PER SERVING 626 kcals, protein 36g, carbs 62g, fat 26g, sat fat 11g, fibre 3g, sugar 16.5g, salt 1.3g

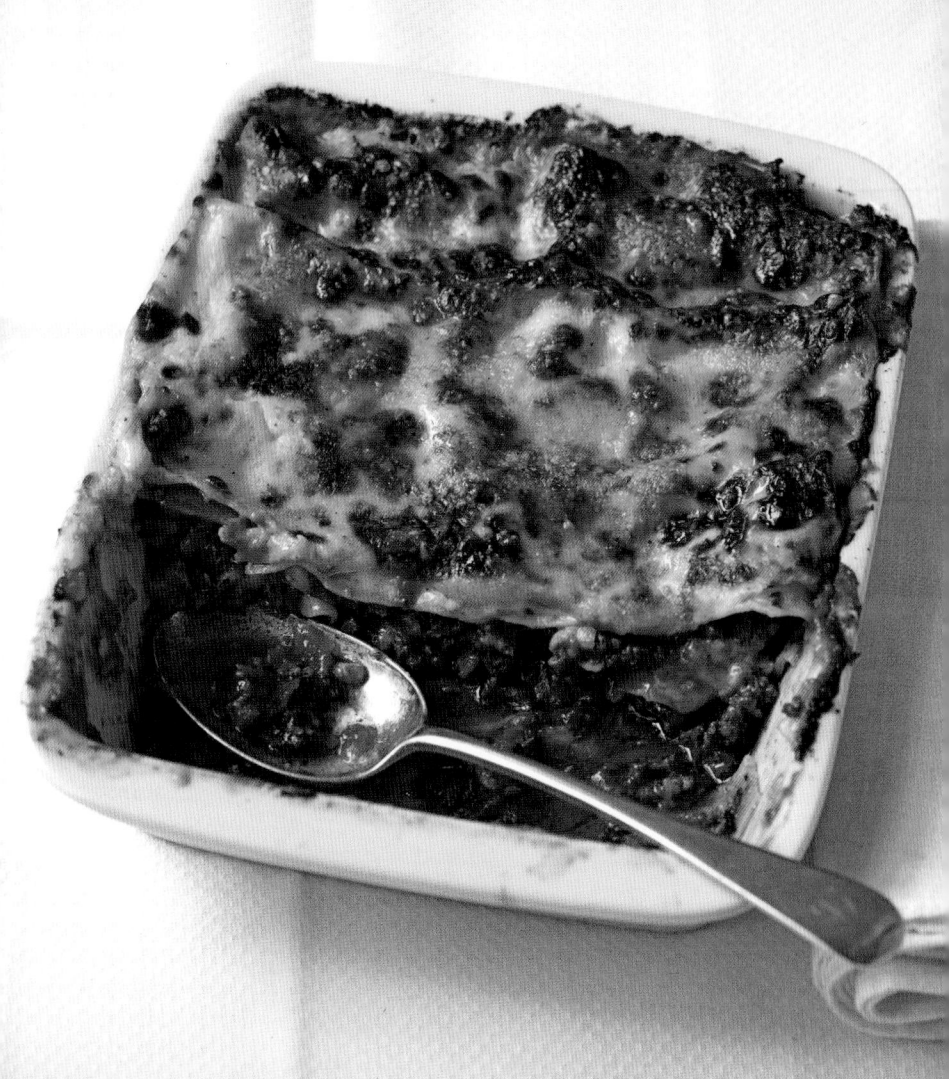

Spaghetti & meatballs

This recipe makes a big batch, but instead of halving the quantities why not make the whole thing, then freeze what you don't need?

TAKES 1 HOUR ● SERVES ABOUT 10

8 gluten-free pork sausages
1kg/2lb 4oz minced beef
1 onion, finely chopped
½ large bunch flat-leaf parsley,
   finely chopped
85g/3oz Parmesan, grated, plus extra
   to garnish (optional)
100g/4oz gluten-free white bread,
   whizzed to crumbs
2 eggs, beaten
olive oil, for roasting
gluten-free spaghetti, (about 85g/3oz
   per portion), to serve

FOR THE SAUCE

3 tbsp olive oil
4 garlic cloves, crushed
4 × 400g cans chopped tomatoes
125ml/4fl oz red wine (optional)
3 tbsp caster sugar
½ large bunch flat-leaf parsley,
   finely chopped
few basil leaves (optional)

1 First make the meatballs. Split the sausage skins and squeeze the meat into a bowl. Add the mince, onion, parsley, Parmesan, crumbs, beaten eggs and seasoning. Get your hands in and mix.
2 Heat oven to 220C/200C fan/gas 7. Roll the mince mixture into about 50 golf-ball-sized meatballs. Set aside any meatballs for freezing, allowing about five per portion, then spread the rest out in a roasting tin. Drizzle with a little oil (about 1 teaspoon per portion), shake to coat, then roast for 20–30 minutes.
3 Meanwhile, make the sauce. Heat the oil in a pan. Add the garlic and sizzle for 1 minute. Stir in the tomatoes, wine, if using, sugar, parsley and some seasoning. Simmer for 15–20 minutes. Stir in the basil leaves, if using, spoon out any sauce for freezing, then add the cooked meatballs to the pan to keep warm while you boil the spaghetti. Spoon the sauce and meatballs over spaghetti and serve with extra Parmesan and a few basil leaves.

PER SERVING 870 kcals, protein 46g, carbs 95g, fat 37g, sat fat 13g, fibre 5g, sugar 13g, salt 1.34g

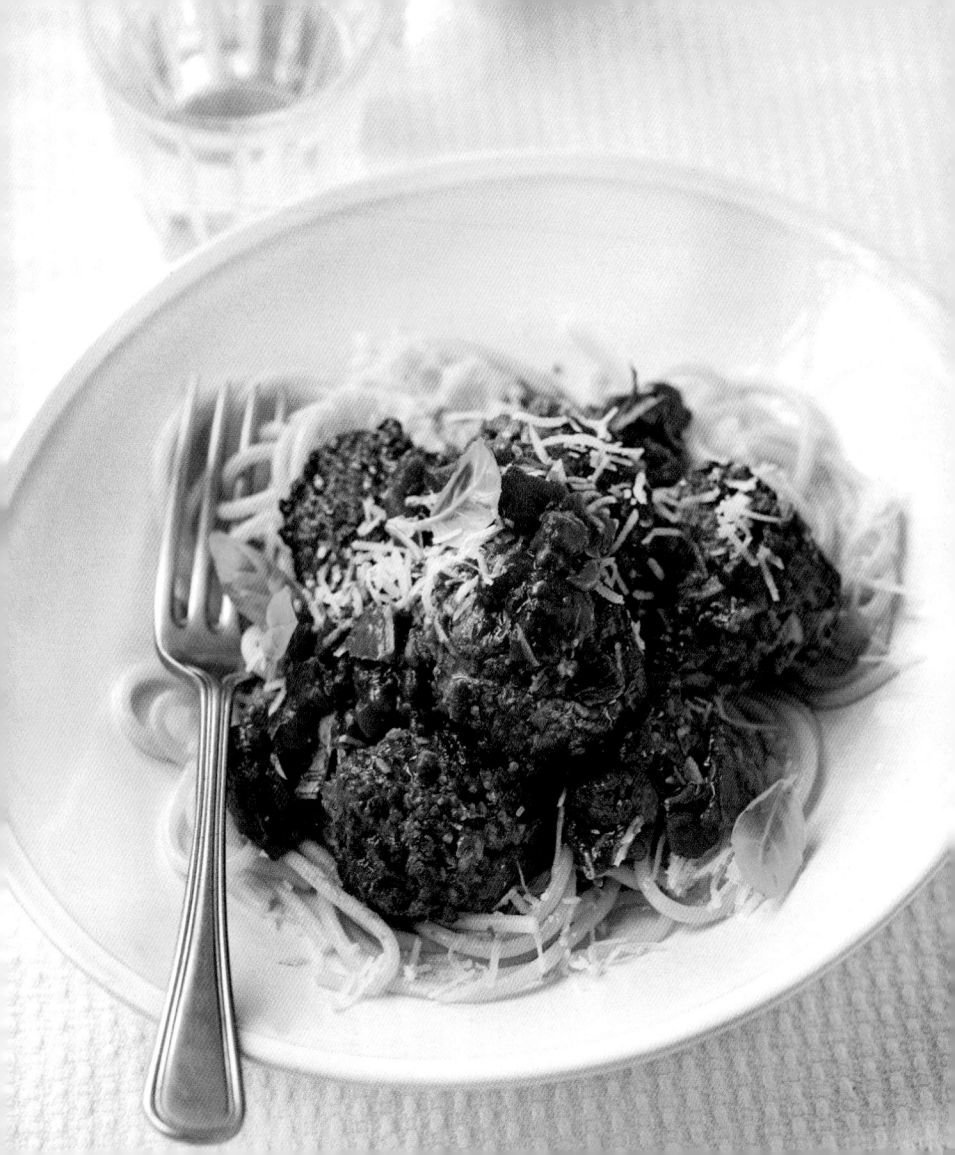

Corn cakes with avocado salsa

Who can resist a corn cake? But if you do fancy a change, swap the corn for a little grated courgette or crispy bacon bits.

TAKES 20 MINUTES • SERVES 2

50g/2oz gluten-free plain flour
½ tsp bicarbonate of soda
1 egg, beaten
200g/7oz canned or frozen sweetcorn
bunch spring onions, trimmed and
    finely chopped
1 avocado, cut into small chunks
1 lime, ½ juiced and ½ cut into
    4 wedges
handful coriander leaves, chopped
1–2 tbsp vegetable oil

1 In a bowl, combine the flour, bicarb, egg, corn and half the onions with some seasoning, then mix well. Mix the avocado with the remaining onions, the lime juice, coriander and some seasoning for the salsa.

2 Heat 1 tablespoon of the oil in a non-stick frying pan. Drop tablespoons of the corn mixture into the frying pan, smoothing them down to form cakes. Cook for about 2–3 minutes on each side over a medium heat, adding the remaining oil, if you need to. Serve hot with the avocado salsa and lime wedges.

PER SERVING 436 kcals, protein 11g, carbs 48g, fat 24g, sat fat 3g, fibre 5g, sugar 11g, salt 1.04g

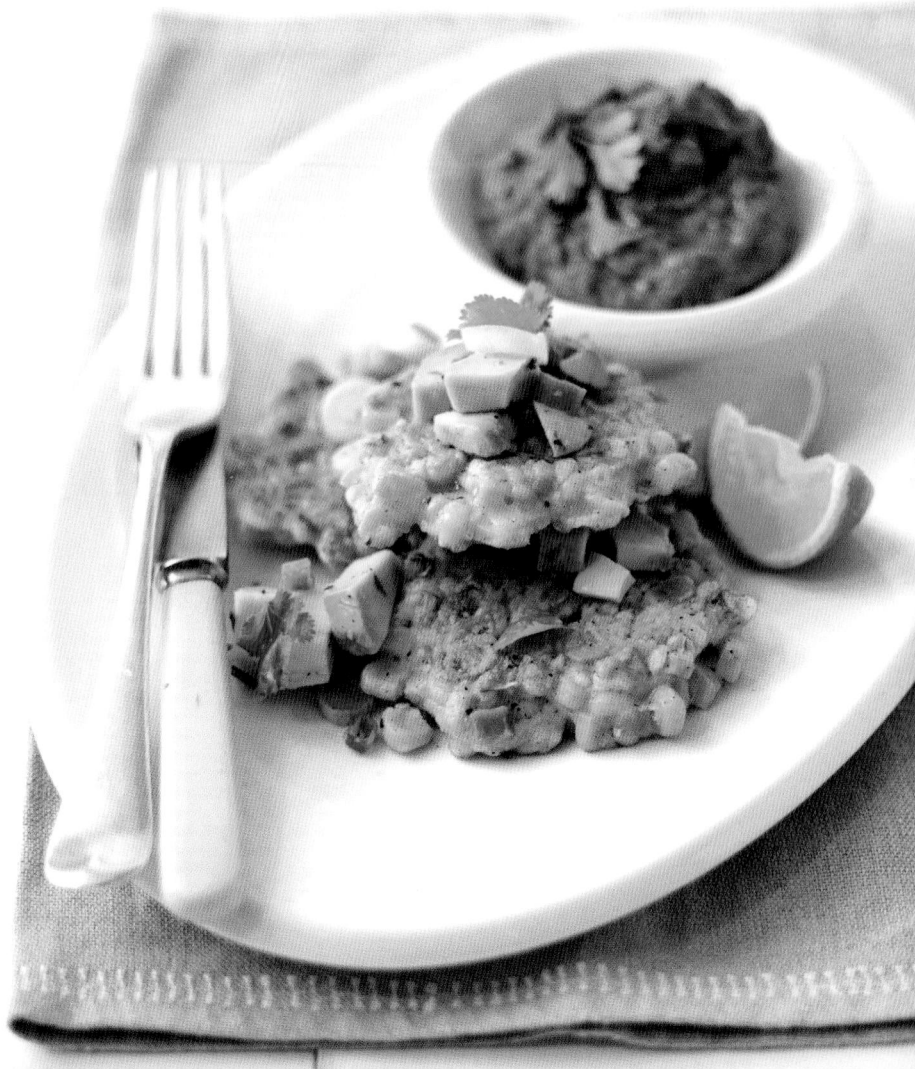

Pizza rolls

Don't waste the roll tops and scooped-out insides from this recipe – make them into breadcrumbs or crunchy croutons for a salad.

TAKES 30 MINUTES ● MAKES 6

6 gluten-free bread rolls
2 tbsp tomato purée
6 slices ham
3 tomatoes, sliced
2 balls mozzarella, sliced
2 tsp dried oregano
6 black olives (optional)
side salad, to serve

1 Heat oven to 180C/160C fan/gas 4. Cut the tops off the rolls and scoop out the insides. Spread the rolls with tomato purée, then fill with ham, tomatoes and finally the mozzarella. Scatter with dried oregano and top each with an olive, if you like.

2 Put the rolls on a baking sheet and bake for 15 minutes until the rolls are crusty brown and the cheese is bubbling. Leave to rest for a minute, then serve hot with a side salad.

PER SERVING 275 kcals, protein 17g, carbs 30g, fat 11g, sat fat 6g, fibre 2g, sugar 4g, salt 1.99g

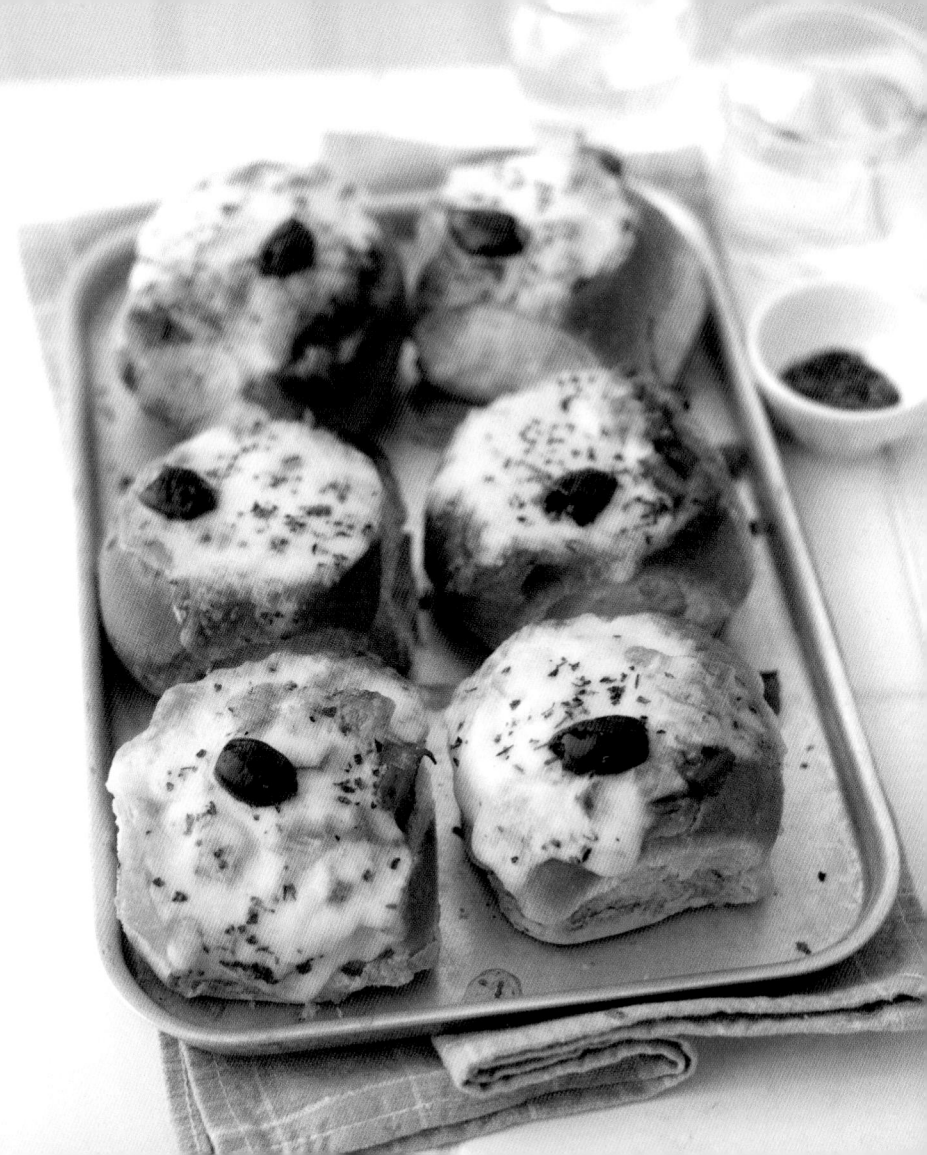

Dippy eggs with Marmite soldiers

An egg with soldiers is the perfect snack any time of the day, for any age! This twist on the classic adds lots of extra goodness without extra fuss.

TAKES 10 MINUTES • SERVES 2

2 large eggs
4 slices gluten-free wholemeal bread
knob of butter
few tsp gluten-free yeast extract (we used Marmite)
25g/1oz mixed seeds

1 Bring a pan of water to a simmer. Add the eggs, simmer for 2 minutes if they are at room temperature, 3 minutes if fridge-cold, then turn off the heat. Cover the pan and leave for 2 minutes more.
2 Meanwhile, toast the bread and spread thinly with butter, then Marmite. To serve, cut into soldiers and dip into the egg, then a few mixed seeds.

PER SERVING 372 kcals, protein 17g, carbs 31g, fat 21g, sat fat 8g, fibre 4g, sugar 2g, salt 1.09g

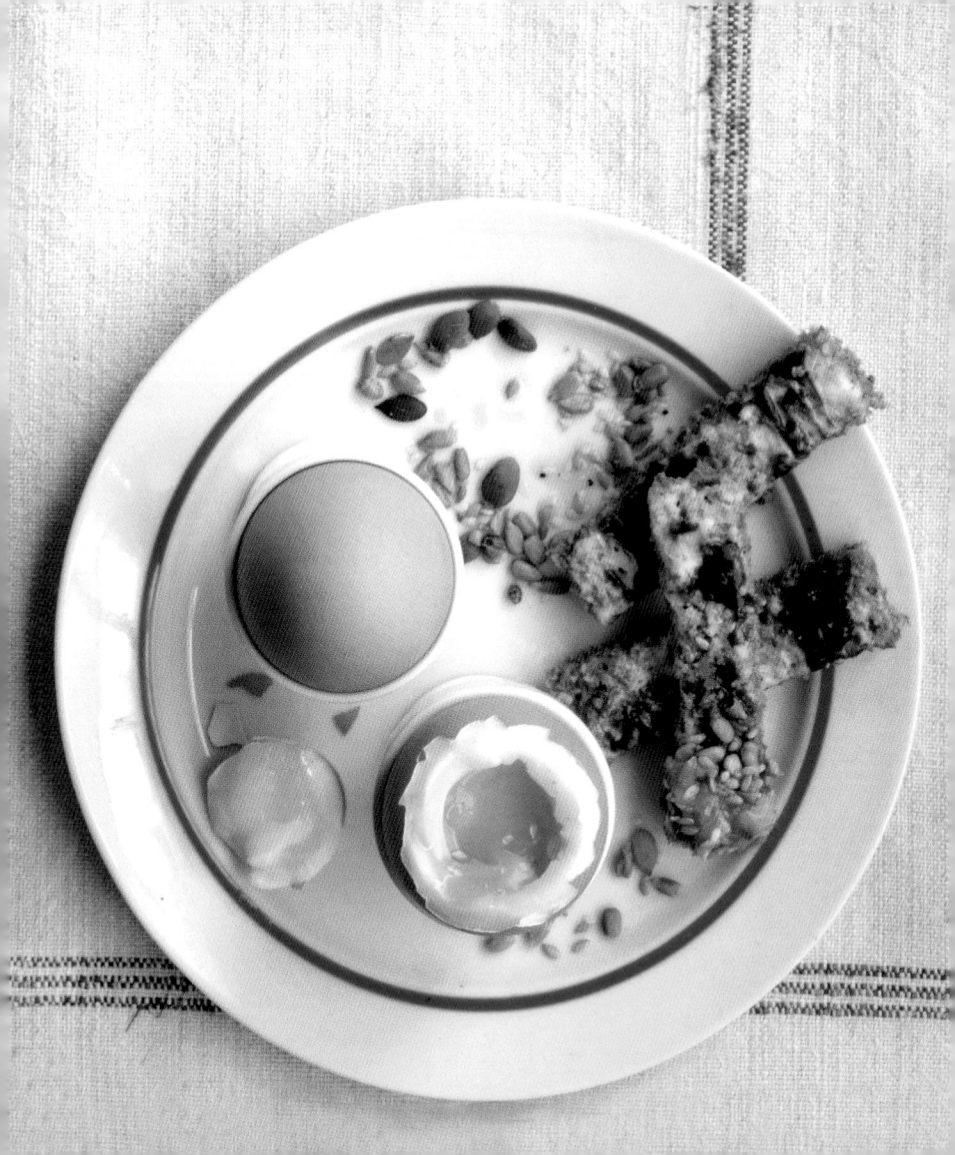

Club sandwich

For a vegetarian alternative, use slices of grilled aubergine and courgette instead of chicken and bacon.

TAKES 20 MINUTES ● SERVES 1

4 rashers streaky bacon
3 slices gluten-free white bread
2 tsp mayo
2 tsp salad cream
1 hard-boiled egg, sliced
1 tomato, sliced
few thick slices chicken or turkey
    breast
small handful salad leaves
handful crisps, to serve (optional)

1 Heat the grill and cook the bacon, turning halfway through, until crisp. Toast the bread. Mix the mayo and salad cream, and spread over one slice of the toasted bread.
2 Layer on the egg, tomato and half of the bacon, then top with another slice of bread. Add the chicken or turkey, the rest of the bacon, then salad leaves. Finish with the final slice of bread and cut into quarters. Secure with cocktail sticks and serve with crisps, if you like.

PER SERVING 744 kcals, protein 62g, carbs 49g, fat 35g, sat fat 10g, fibre 2g, sugar 6g, salt 5.81g

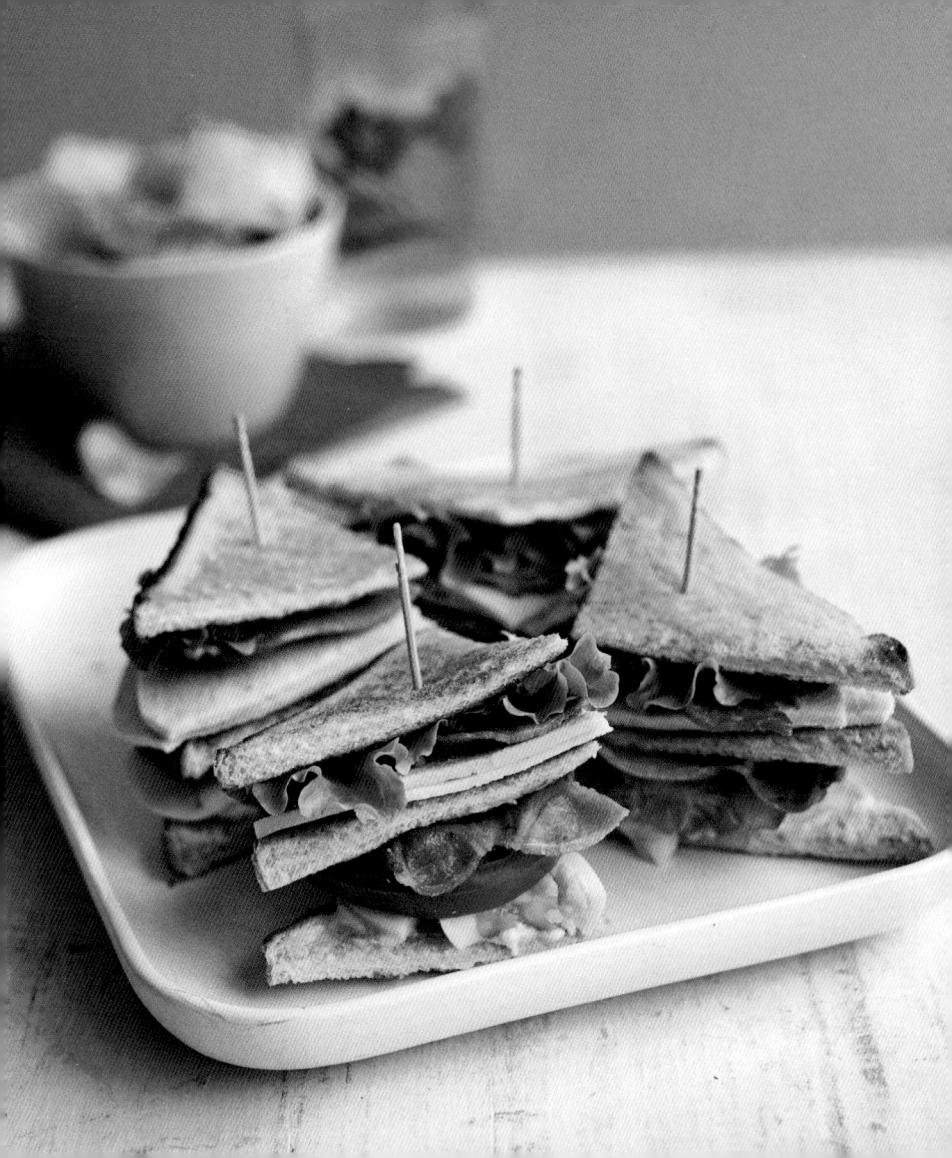

Chicken nachos

Get the kids to layer up this dish, then quickly bake before letting everyone dive in!

TAKES 15 MINUTES ● SERVES 4

200g/7oz gluten-free plain tortilla chips

2 cooked chicken breasts, shredded
  into small pieces

6 spring onions, thinly sliced

140g/5oz Red Leicester, grated

1 small jar red or green sliced pickled
  jalapeños

small bunch coriander, leaves roughly
  chopped, to garnish

your choice of salsa, hot pepper sauce,
  crème fraîche, guacamole or extra
  jalapeños, to serve

1 Heat oven to 200C/180C fan/gas 6.
Layer up the tortilla chips in an
ovenproof dish or baking sheet with the
shredded chicken, spring onions, cheese
and pickled jalapeños.

2 Bake for 8 minutes or until the cheese
is melted. To serve, sprinkle with the
coriander and eat with your favourite
accompaniments.

PER SERVING 484 kcals, protein 31g, carbs 35g,
fat 25g, sat fat 8g, fibre 3g, sugar 5g, salt 2.2g

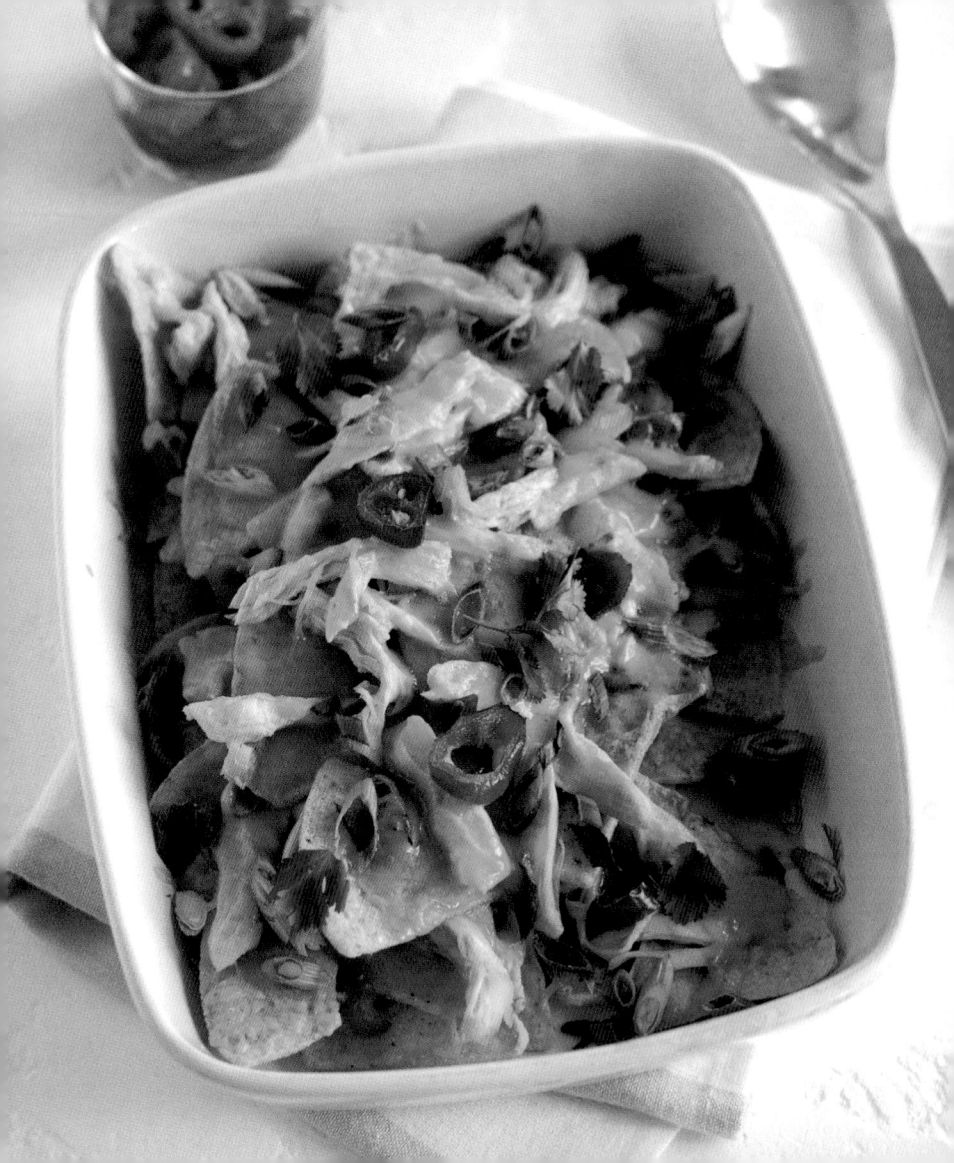

Red onion & Indian spiced houmous

Keep homemade houmous in a tub in the fridge, and you can dip in anytime you get the munchies.

TAKES 25 MINUTES • SERVES 2

2 tbsp olive oil
1 red onion, thinly sliced
1 tsp each cumin seeds and coriander
    seeds
½ tsp fennel seeds
1 × 400g can chickpeas, rinsed and
    drained
juice ½ lemon
1 tbsp tahini paste
2 tsp finely chopped coriander
gluten-free pitta breads, to serve

1 In a non-stick pan heat 1 tablespoon of the oil, then fry the onion until soft and lightly browned. Remove from the heat and set aside to cool while you prepare the rest of the ingredients.
2 Toast the spices for a couple of minutes on a low heat, then remove from the heat and grind to make a powder. In a food processor, blitz together the chickpeas, lemon juice, tahini, spices, some salt, the chopped coriander and cooled red onion until smooth.
3 Tip into a serving bowl and dress with the remaining olive oil. Warm the pitta breads and serve alongside the houmous.

PER SERVING 314 kcals, protein 11g, carbs 25g, fat 20g, sat fat 2g, fibre 6g, sugar 4g, salt 0.69g

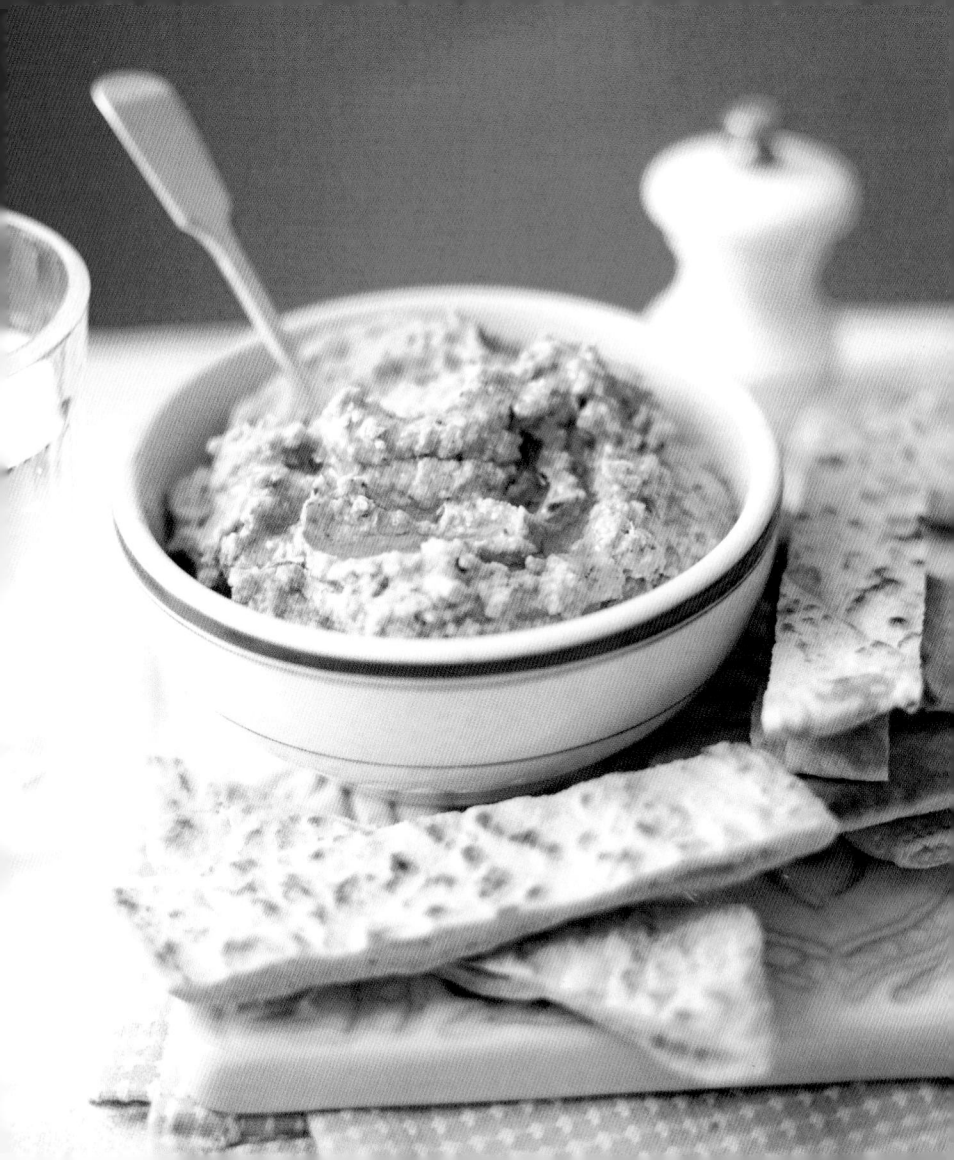

Sticky popcorn pots

Popcorn is a great gluten-free snack just as it is, but the trend now is for fancy flavours; so why not treat yours to a yummy coating of homemade caramel.

TAKES 10 MINUTES • SERVES 12

50g/2oz popping corn
140g/5oz salted butter
140g/5oz light muscovado sugar

1 Pop the popping corn according to the pack instructions.

2 Meanwhile, melt the butter in a pan, then tip in the sugar. Heat gently until the sugar has dissolved. Pour the caramel over the popcorn and stir to coat. Cool, then serve in plastic cups.

PER SERVING 192 kcals, protein 2g, carbs 25g, fat 10g, sat fat 6g, fibre 1g, sugar 12g, salt 0.01g

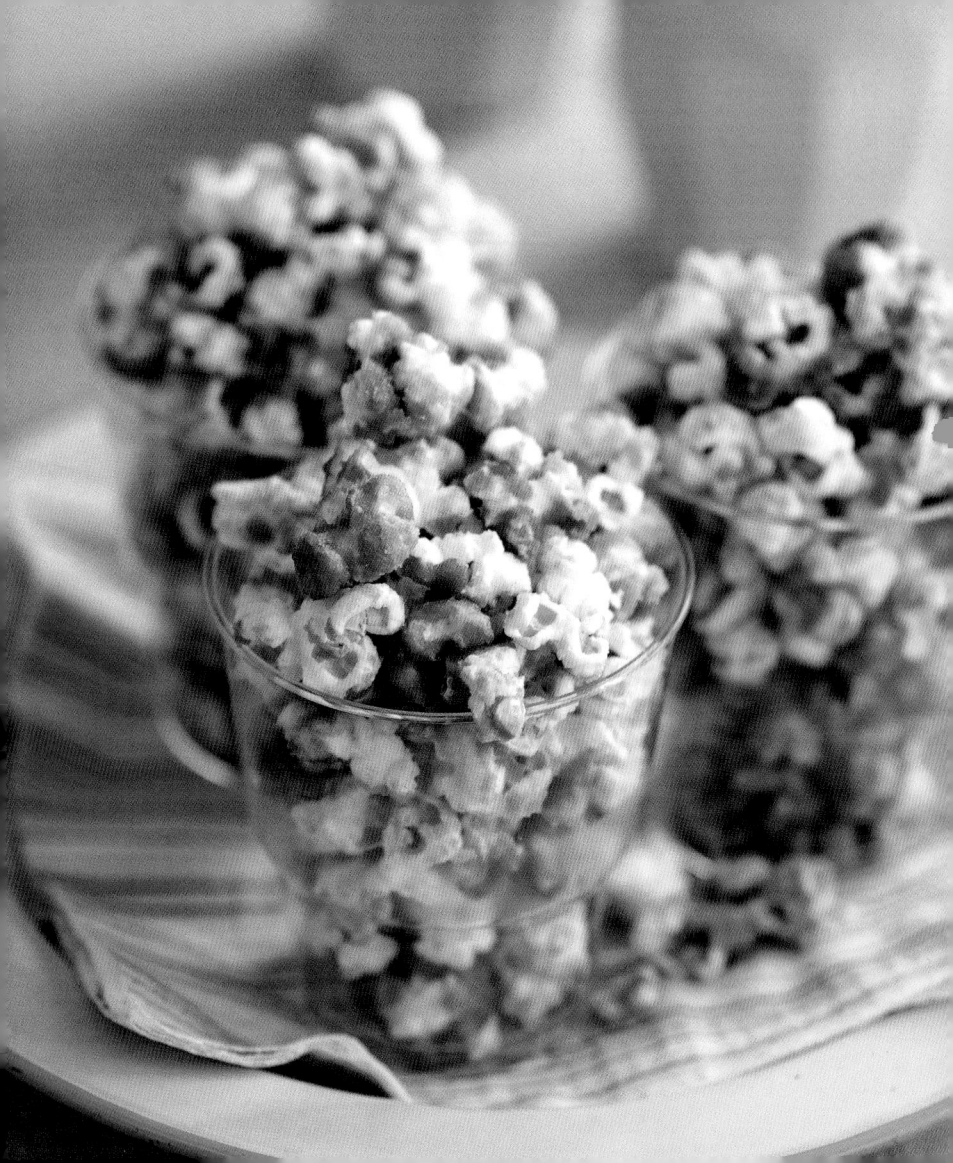

Fruity fondue

This is a fun way to get the kids to eat more fruit. On weekends make it even more of a treat by alternating the fruit with marshmallows.

TAKES 15 MINUTES ● SERVES 4

650g/1lb 7oz mixed fruits, such as
  strawberries, pineapple chunks,
  grapes, mango chunks, melon
  chunks
100g/4oz milk chocolate
150g pot fat-free yogurt (use your
  favourite flavour)

1 Thread the fruits on to wooden skewers.

2 Melt the milk chocolate on a low heat in the microwave, then transfer to a small serving bowl. Serve the fruit kebabs on a platter with the yogurt and melted chocolate in small bowls for dipping and get everyone to dig in.

PER SERVING 216 kcals, protein 5g, carbs 33g, fat 8g, sat fat 5g, fibre 2g, sugar 33g, salt 0.16g

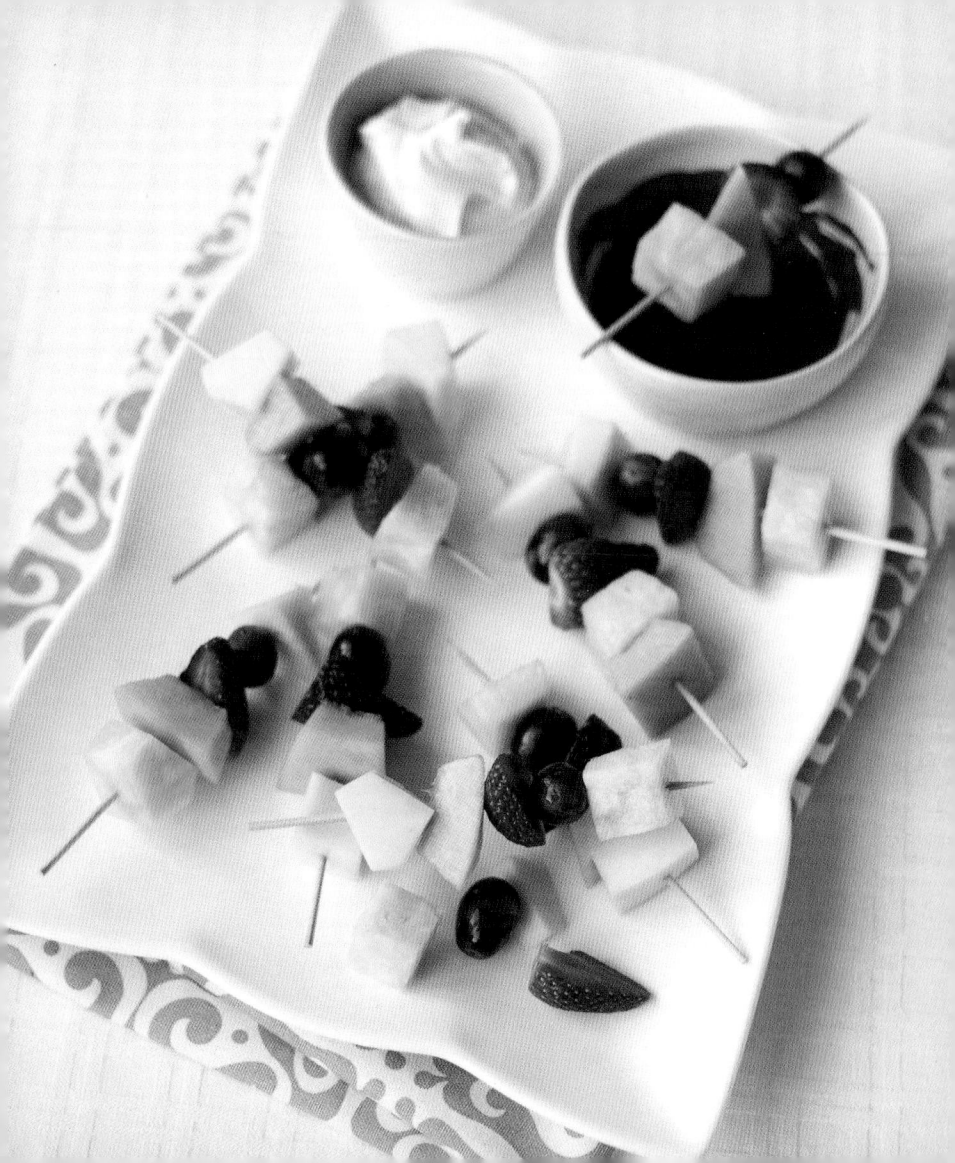

Buckwheat pancakes

The thin versions are perfect for Pancake Day, but, let's face it, on every other day of the year you can't beat a fat American-style pancake smothered in maple syrup.

TAKES 35 MINUTES • SERVES 4–6

4 tbsp golden caster sugar

140g/5oz buckwheat flour

85g/3oz gluten-free plain flour

2 tsp cinnamon

1 tsp bicarbonate of soda

3 eggs

284ml pot buttermilk

few knobs of butter

yogurt and berries, or maple syrup,
   to serve

1 Mix the sugar, flours, cinnamon and bicarb in a large bowl. Make a well in the centre and crack in the eggs. Gradually whisk in with the buttermilk to make a smooth batter.

2 Melt a knob of butter in a non-stick frying pan. Add spoonfuls of batter to make pancakes about 8–10cm/3–4in wide. Cook for a couple of minutes until set on the bottom and bubbles appear on the surface, then flip and cook the other side. Keep the pancakes warm in a low oven while you finish up the batter. Serve two or three per person, with your favourite toppings.

PER SERVING 504 kcals, protein 14g, carbs 85g, fat 15g, sat fat 7g, fibre 3g, sugar 38g, salt 1.28g

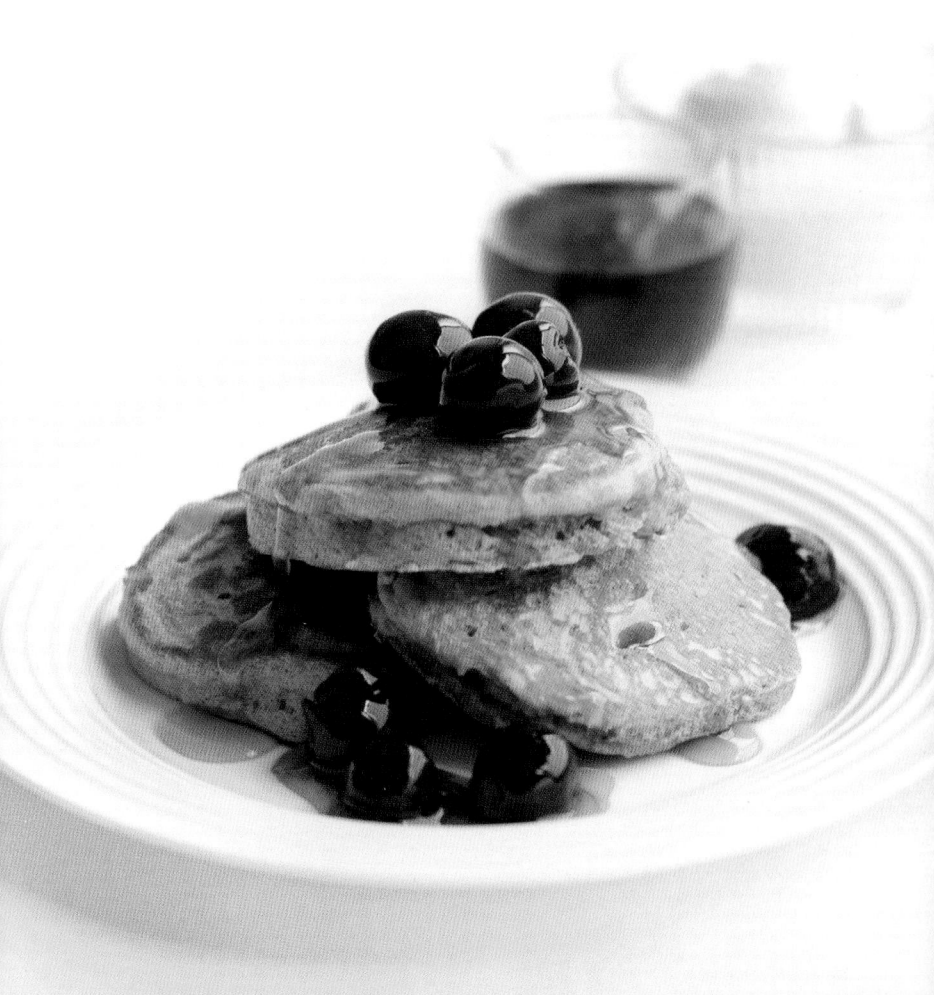

Triple cheese & onion muffins

These muffins are delicious freshly baked and smothered with butter. Keep leftovers in an airtight tin and refresh in the microwave before eating.

TAKES 50 MINUTES • MAKES 12

150ml/¼ pint sunflower oil, plus extra
   for greasing
1 large egg
284ml pot buttermilk
150ml/5½fl oz milk
500g/1lb 2oz gluten-free self-raising
   flour
1 tsp English mustard powder
140g/5oz grated mature Cheddar
1 bunch spring onions, sliced
small bunch chives, snipped
200g/7oz full-fat soft cheese, gently
   diced into 1–2cm/½–¾in cubes
25g/1oz Parmesan (or vegetarian
   alternative), grated

1 Heat oven to 200C/180C fan/gas 6 and grease a 12-hole muffin tin. Whisk the oil, egg, buttermilk and milk. Mix the flour, 1 teaspoon salt and the mustard powder in a mixing bowl, then mix in the Cheddar, spring onions and chives.
2 Use a large spoon to fold the wet mixture into the dry, don't over mix just lightly combine, and with the last few folds mix in the soft cheese cubes. Divide the mixture among the tins, scatter with Parmesan and bake for 25 minutes.

PER MUFFIN 389 kcals, protein 9g, carbs 35g, fat 24g, sat fat 8g, fibre 0.7g, sugar 2g, salt 0.9g

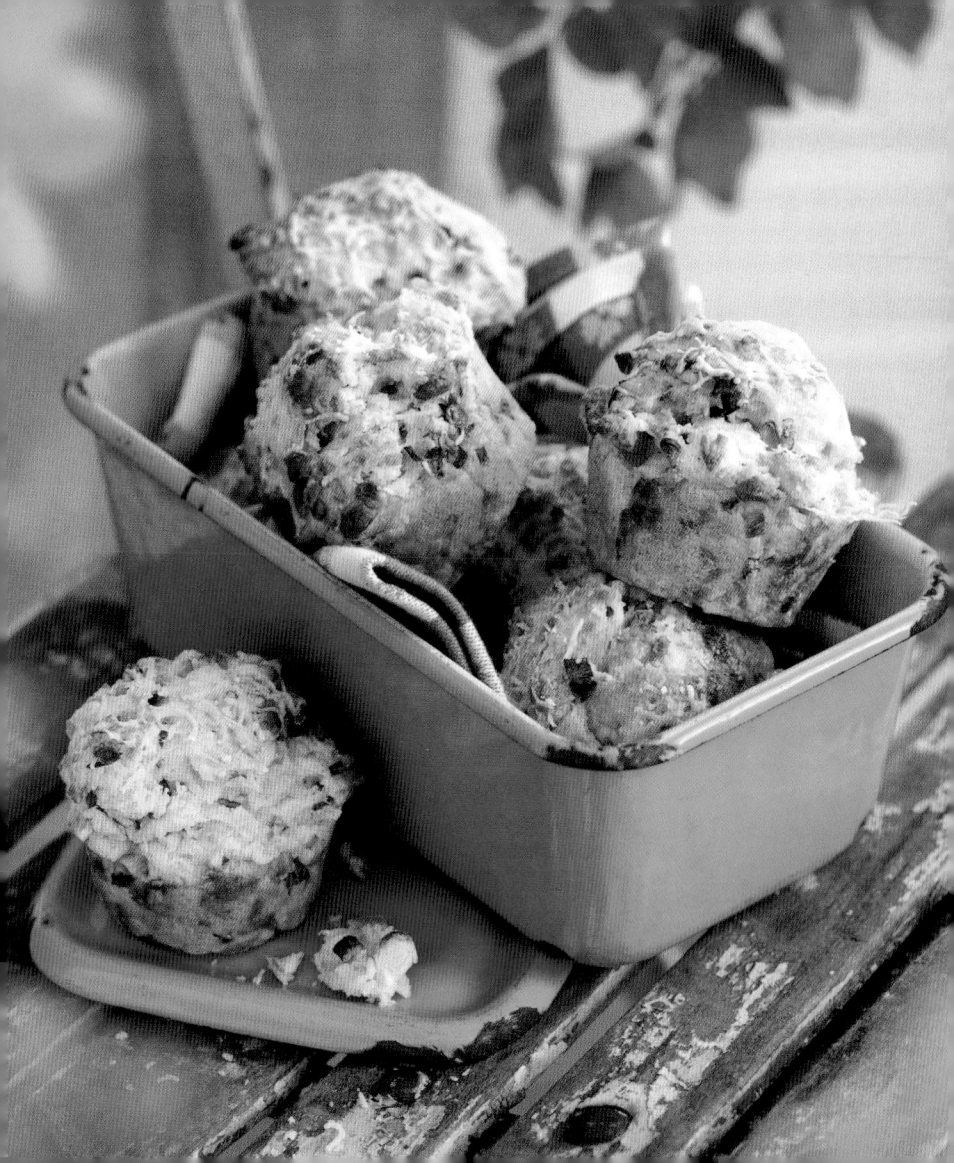

Macadamia & cranberry American cookies

These are completely irresistible and a great recipe for the kids to help you make.

TAKES ABOUT 45 MINUTES
- **MAKES 55**

3 × 200g bars white chocolate, chopped
200g/7oz butter
2 eggs
100g/4oz light muscovado sugar
175g/6oz golden caster sugar
2 tsp vanilla extract
350g/12oz gluten-free plain flour
2 tsp gluten-free baking powder
1 tsp ground cinnamon
100g/4oz dried cranberries
100g/4oz macadamia nuts, chopped

1 Heat oven to 180C/160C fan/gas 4. Melt 175g/6oz of the chocolate in a bowl set over a pan of simmering water, then allow to cool. Beat in the butter, eggs, sugars and vanilla, preferably with an electric hand whisk, until creamy. Stir in the flour, baking powder, cinnamon and cranberries with two-thirds of the remaining chocolate and macadamias, to make a stiff dough.

2 Using a tablespoon or a small ice-cream scoop, drop small mounds on to a large baking dish, spacing them well apart, then poke in the reserved chocolate and nuts. Bake in batches for 12 minutes until pale golden, leave to harden for 1–2 minutes, then cool on a wire rack.

PER COOKIE 149 kcals, protein 2g, carb 18g, fat 8g, sat fat 4g, fibre none, sugar 13g, salt 0.14g

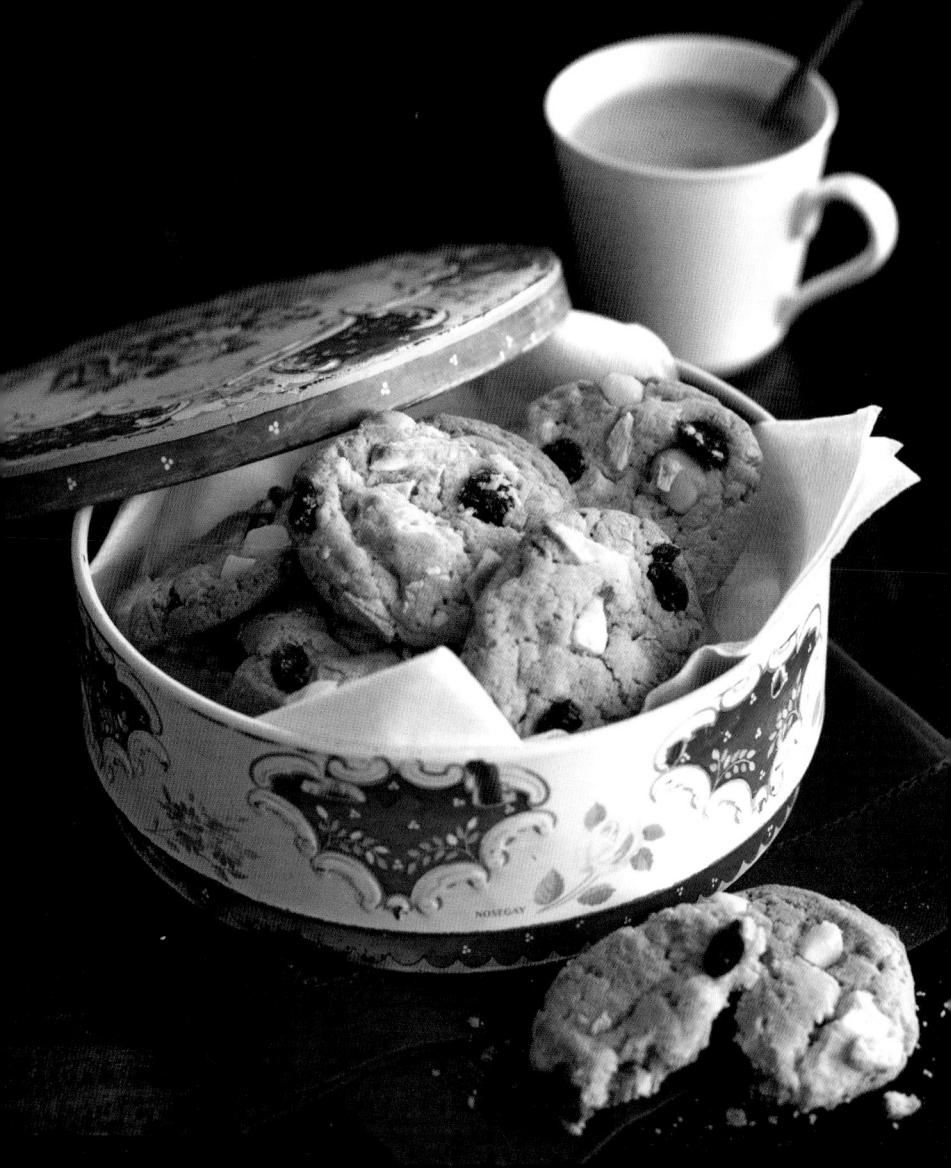

Apricot, honey & pistachio bars

Flapjacks are a great snack as oats release energy slowly so these will keep you full until suppertime.

TAKES 50 MINUTES • MAKES 16

140g/5oz butter
140g/5oz soft brown sugar
2 tbsp honey
175g/6oz gluten-free rolled oats
85g/3oz shelled pistachio nuts, chopped
140g/5oz dried apricots, chopped

1 Put the butter, soft brown sugar and honey in a small pan, then heat gently until melted. Tip the oats, chopped pistachios and chopped apricots into a medium bowl. Pour over the melted butter mixture and stir to combine.

2 Transfer to a 20cm-square greased and lined baking tin and cook at 160C/140C fan/gas 3 for 35–40 minutes. Remove and cool in the tin, then slice into 16 bars. Will keep in an airtight container for up to 4 days.

PER FLAPJACK 193 kcals, protein 3g, carbs 22g, fat 11g, sat fat 5g, fibre 2g, sugar 15g, salt 0.13g

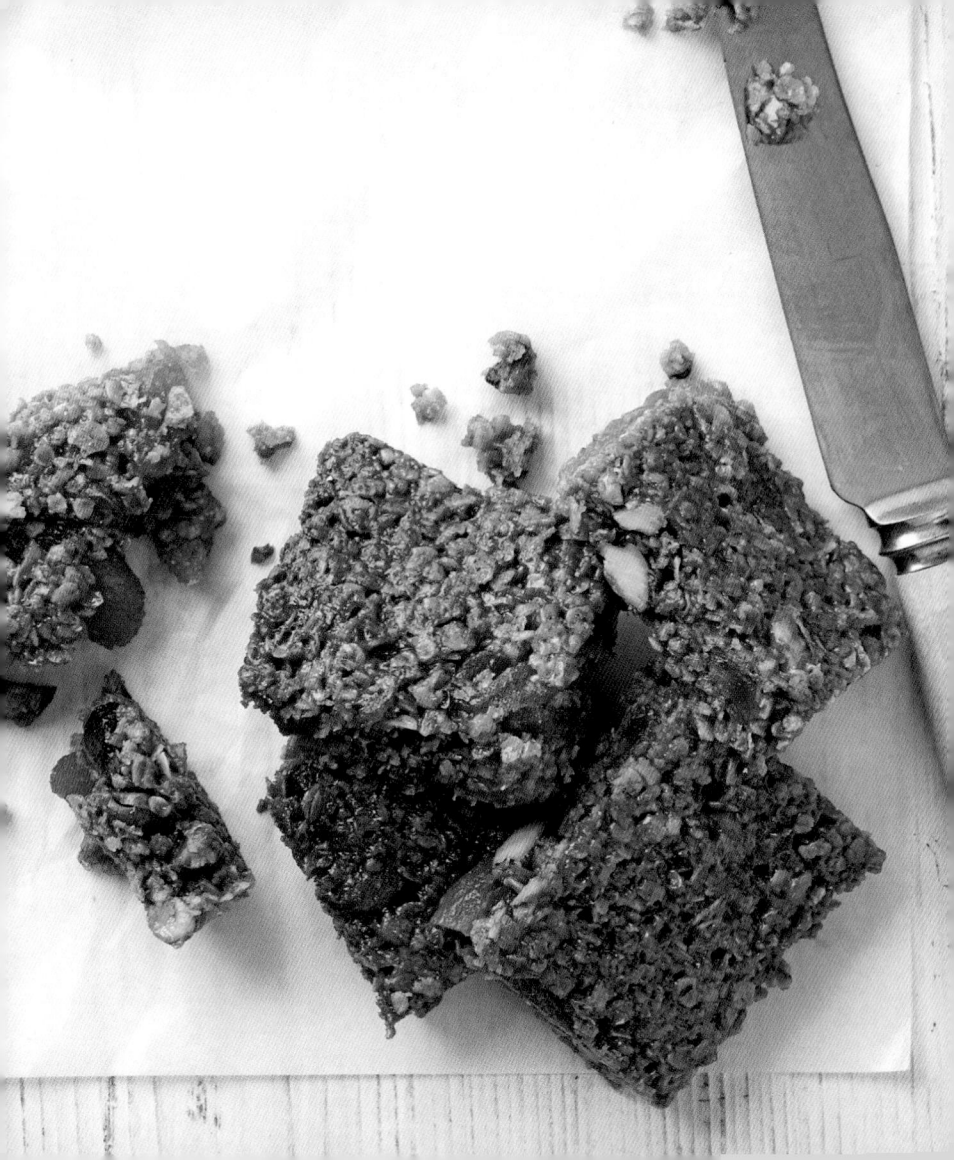

Iced ginger shortcake

These taste pretty good as they are, but even better with a cup of tea and your feet up!

TAKES 50 MINUTES • MAKES 16

175g/6oz butter, plus extra for greasing
85g/3oz caster sugar
100g/4oz gluten-free plain flour
1 tsp xanthan gum
100g/4oz ground rice
2 tsp ground ginger

FOR THE ICING AND DECORATION

100g/4oz butter
2 tbsp golden syrup
8 heaped tbsp icing sugar
2 tsp ground ginger
crystallised ginger, roughly chopped

1 Heat oven to 160C/140C fan/gas 3. Grease a 20cm-square baking tin. Beat the butter and sugar until pale and fluffy. Add in the flour, xanthan gum, ground rice and ginger, then mix together with a knife. Using lightly floured hands, bring the mixture together to form a dough, then spread it into the greased baking tin. Bake for 30 minutes until golden. Remove from the oven and leave to cool slightly.

2 For the icing, melt the butter and syrup in a pan. Remove from the heat, sift in the icing sugar and ginger, then mix until smooth and glossy. Cool until almost cold and beat well again. Spread the icing over the shortcake using a palette knife, decorate with chopped crystallised ginger then cut into 16 slices.

PER SHORTCAKE 249 kcals, protein 2g, carbs 31g, fat 14g, sat fat 9g, fibre none, sugar 21g, salt 0.28g

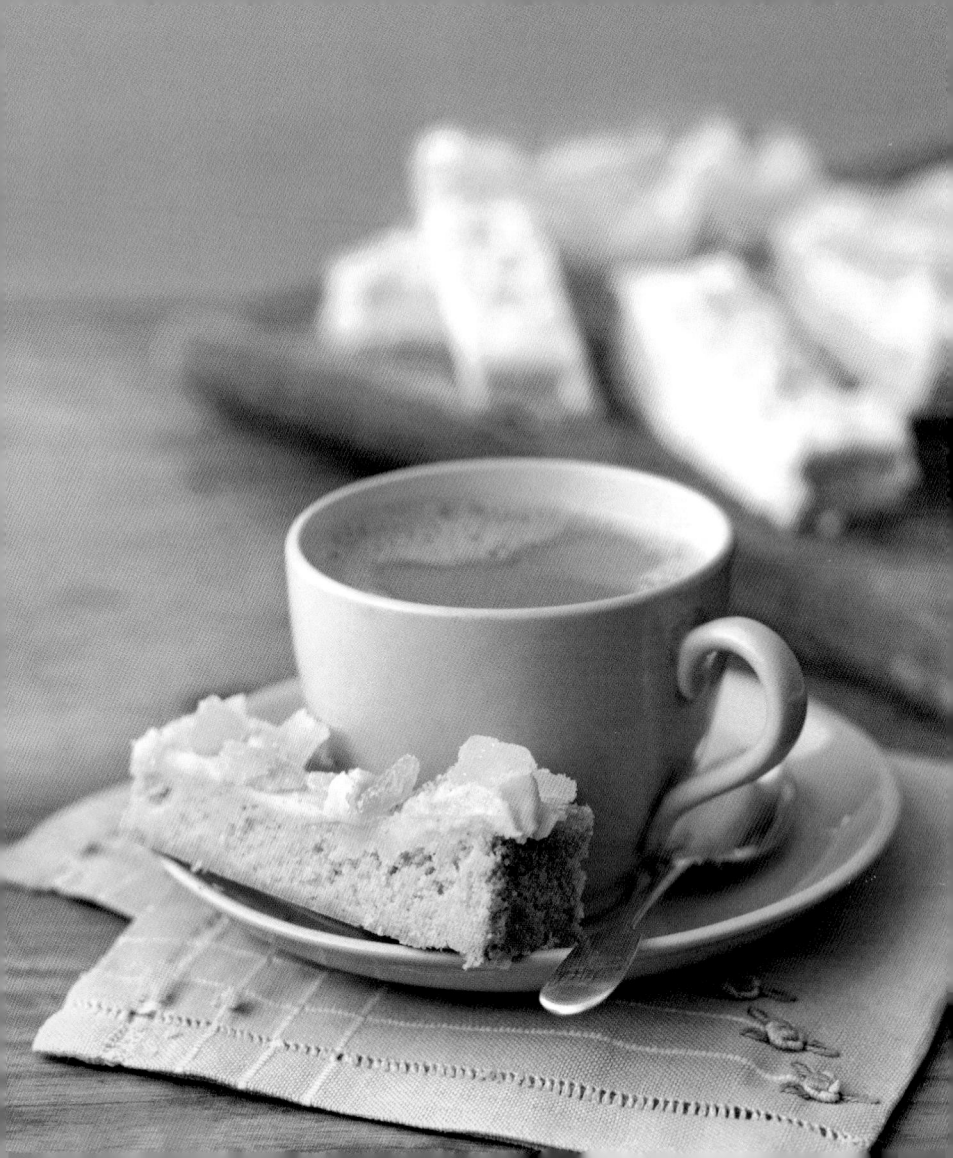

Super berry smoothie

If you make your own smoothies rather than buying ready-made, you can make sure you know exactly what goes into them – so there are no nasty surprises!

TAKES 10 MINUTES • SERVES 4

450g bag frozen berries, defrosted
450g pot fat-free strawberry yogurt
100ml/4fl oz milk
25g/1oz gluten-free porridge oats
2 tsp clear honey, to drizzle (optional)

1 Whizz the berries, yogurt, milk and oats together in a blender until smooth. Pour into four glasses and serve with a drizzle of honey, if you like.

PER SERVING 117 kcals, protein 8g, carbs 18g, fat 1g, sat fat 1g, fibre 4g, sugar 14g, salt 0.2g

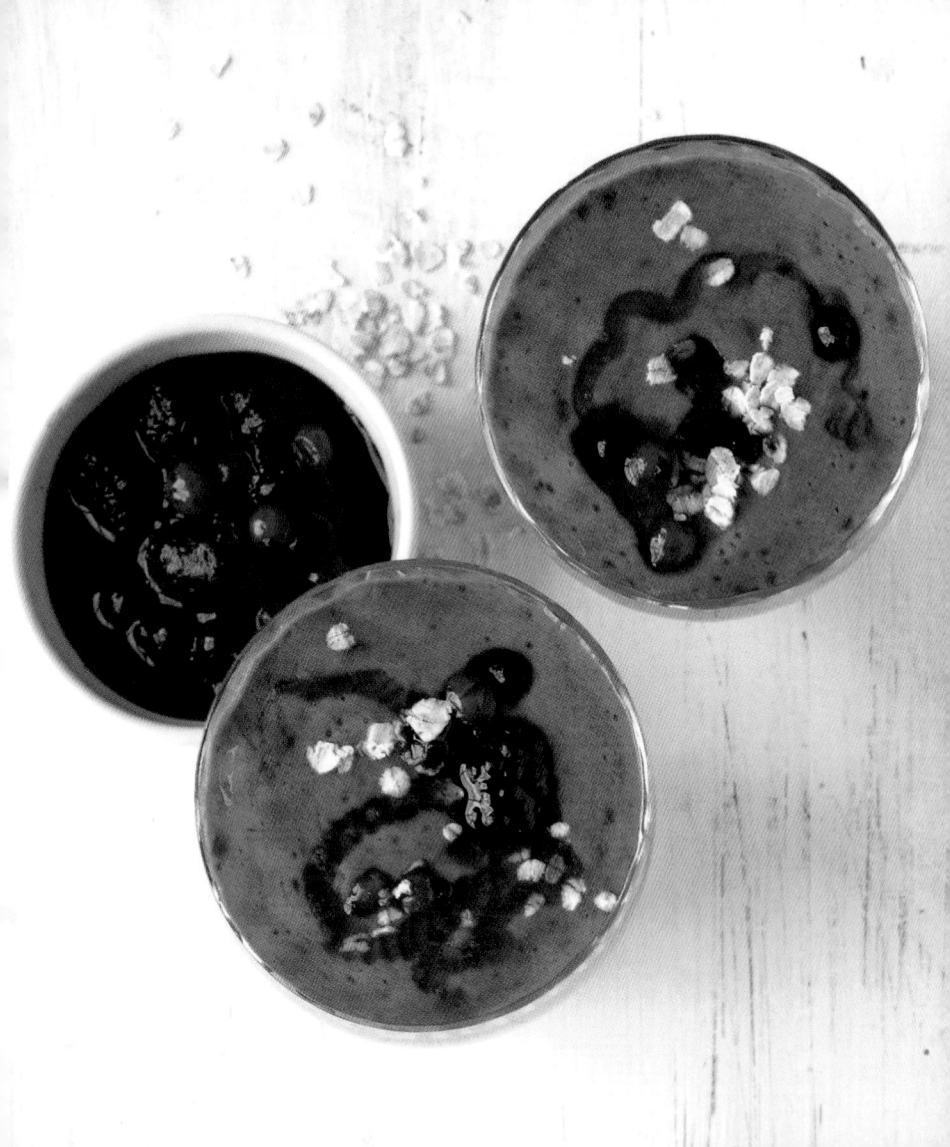

Bitter orange & poppy seed cake

Toasting poppy seeds in a dry pan for a few minutes really brings out their nutty flavour.

TAKES 1½ HOURS

- **CUTS INTO 8 SLICES**

175g/6oz butter, softened, plus extra
    for greasing
3 tbsp good-quality thick-cut
    marmalade
150g pot natural yogurt
3 eggs
175g/6oz golden caster sugar
100g/4oz gluten-free self-raising flour
    (add 1 tsp xanthan gum if it doesn't
    contain any)
100g/4oz polenta
½ tsp gluten-free baking powder
zest 1 orange
2 tsp poppy seeds, toasted

FOR THE STICKY TOPPING

juice ½ orange
5 tbsp marmalade

1 Heat oven to 160C/140C fan/gas 3. Butter a 900g loaf tin. Line the base and sides with baking parchment. Heat the marmalade in a pan until melted. Beat in the yogurt, then cool for a few minutes.

2 Put the remaining cake ingredients into a bowl and beat with an electric whisk until smooth. Quickly beat in the marmalade mix, then pour into the tin. Leave the mix mounded in the middle rather than levelling the top, to help it rise and crack in the middle.

3 Bake for 1 hour – 1 hour 10 minutes until golden and well risen; a skewer should come out clean. Look at the cake after 45 minutes; if it has taken on a lot of colour, loosely cover with baking paper.

4 Meanwhile make the topping. Heat the juice and marmalade in a small pan until the marmalade melts. Set aside to cool, stirring now and again, until you have a thick, but still runny, glaze. Cool the cake in the tin for 10 minutes, then turn on to a wire rack. Spoon the topping over the cake while it is just warm.

PER SLICE 422 kcals, protein 6g, carbs 54g, fat 21g, sat fat 12g, fibre 1g, sugar 35g, salt 0.80g

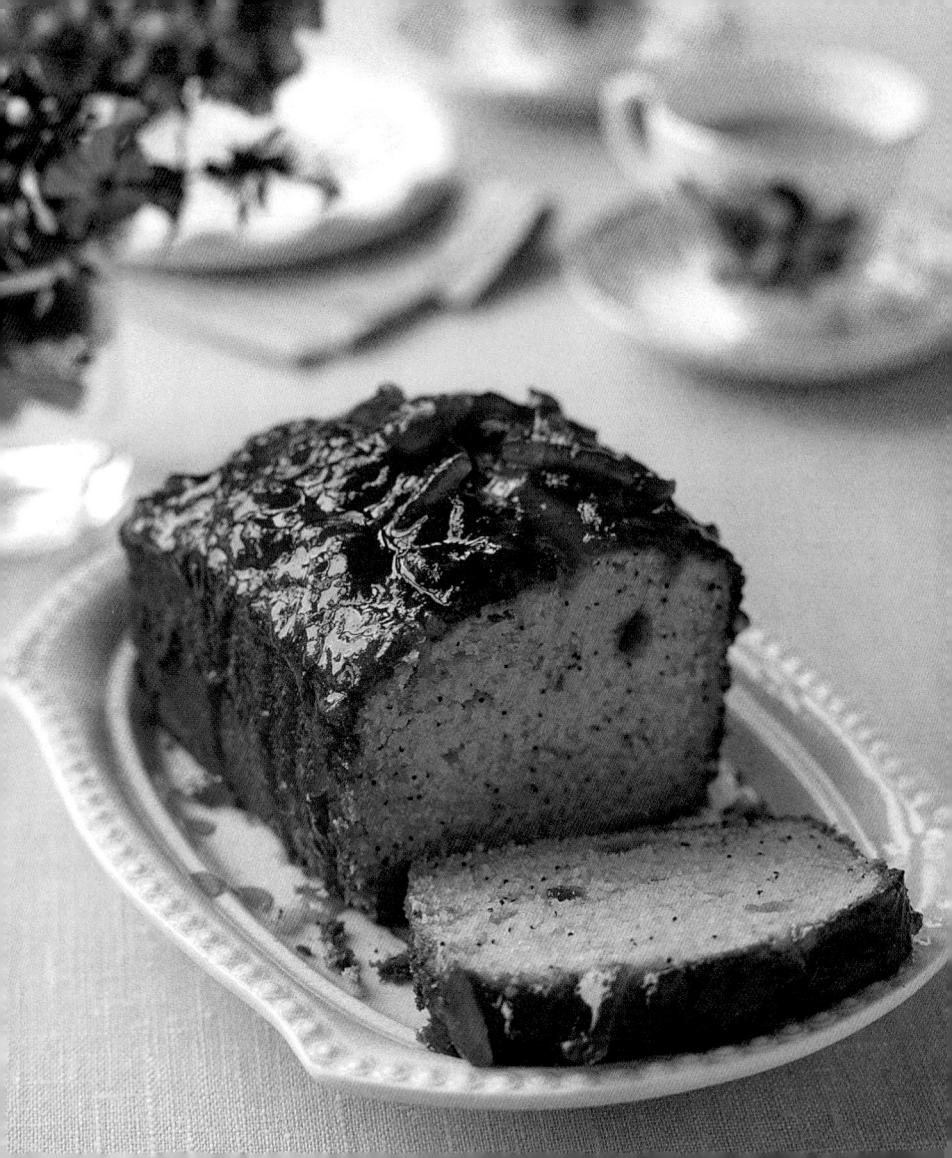

Classic Victoria sponge

You can knock up this classic afternoon tea cake really quickly, and once you've mastered it the fillings and flavour combinations are endless.

TAKES 40 MINUTES, PLUS COOLING
- **CUTS INTO 8–10 SLICES**

200g/7oz unsalted butter, softened, plus extra for greasing
200g/7oz caster sugar
1 tsp vanilla extract
4 medium eggs
140g/5oz gluten-free plain flour
85g/3oz ground almonds
2 tsp xanthan gum
2 tsp gluten-free baking powder
about 6 tbsp raspberry jam
250ml/9fl oz double cream
1 tbsp icing sugar, sifted, plus extra for dusting

1 Heat oven to 190C/170C fan/gas 5. Grease two 20cm-round sandwich tins and line the bases with baking parchment. Put the butter, sugar and vanilla extract into a bowl and beat well to a creamy consistency. Slowly beat in the eggs, one by one, then fold in the flour, ground almonds, xanthan gum and baking powder, and mix well.

2 Divide the mix between the cake tins, put into the oven and bake for about 20 minutes until risen and golden brown. The cakes should spring back when gently pushed in the middle. When ready, remove from the oven and allow to cool for 5 minutes in the tin, before turning out on to a wire rack and cooling completely.

3 Spread the jam onto one cake. Whisk the cream and icing sugar until thick, then spread over the jam. Sandwich the cakes together and dust with icing sugar.

PER SLICE (8) 599 kcals, protein 6g, carbs 56g, fat 40g, sat fat 23g, fibre 1g, sugar 38g, salt 0.35g

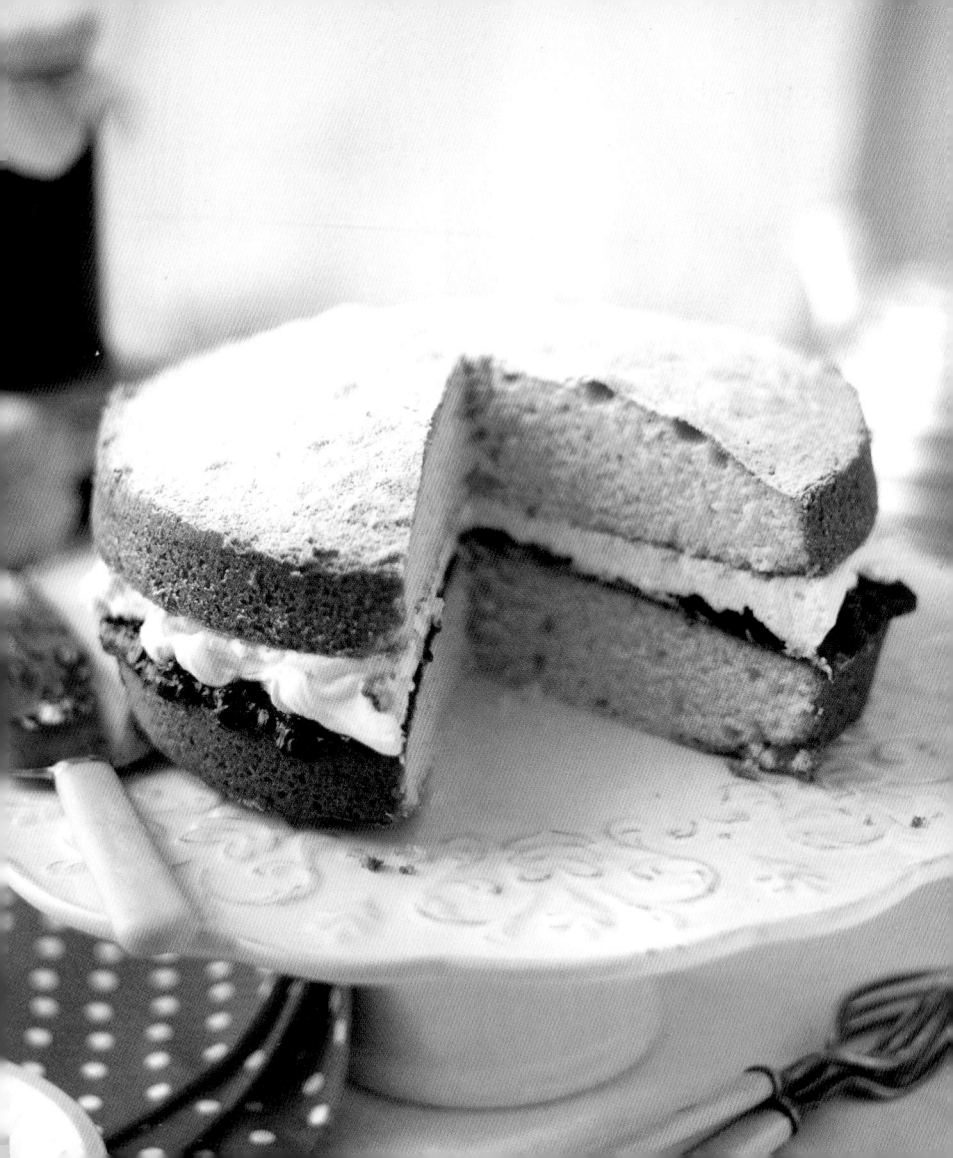

Chestnut truffle cake

This rich cake makes a perfect dinner-party dessert, and it's make-ahead so it'll make entertaining even easier.

TAKES 40 MINUTES, PLUS CHILLING
- **SERVES 6–8**

400g/14oz cooked chestnuts
100g/4oz caster sugar
100g/4oz cold butter, chopped into cubes, plus extra for greasing
100g/4oz dark chocolate, minimum 70% cocoa solids, broken into pieces
3 tbsp milk
1 tsp vanilla extract
2 tbsp cognac

FOR THE TOPPING

100g/4oz dark chocolate, minimum 70% cocoa solids
25g/1oz butter
1 tbsp single cream, plus extra to serve
icing sugar, to dust

1 Put the chestnuts in a food processor with the sugar, then process until fairly smooth. Put the butter and chocolate in a pan with the milk, then gently heat, stirring, until they have melted to a smooth sauce. Stir in the vanilla and cognac. Add to the chestnut mix in the food processor, then whizz again until fairly smooth.

2 Line a lightly buttered small loaf tin with cling film, then pour in the chestnut truffle mix. Smooth the top, then cover the tin with cling film. Chill for 24 hours.

3 To serve, turn out the truffle cake on to a flat plate or board. Peel off the cling film. Gently melt the chocolate, butter and cream for the topping, then spread over the top and sides of the cake. Return to the fridge to set. Will keep in the fridge for another 6 days.

4 Decorate with a dusting of icing sugar. Serve cut into thin slices with a little single cream poured around (cold vanilla custard is also very good).

PER SERVING (6) 525 kcals, protein 4g, carbs 64g, fat 29g, sat fat 17g, fibre 4g, sugar 44g, salt 0.36g

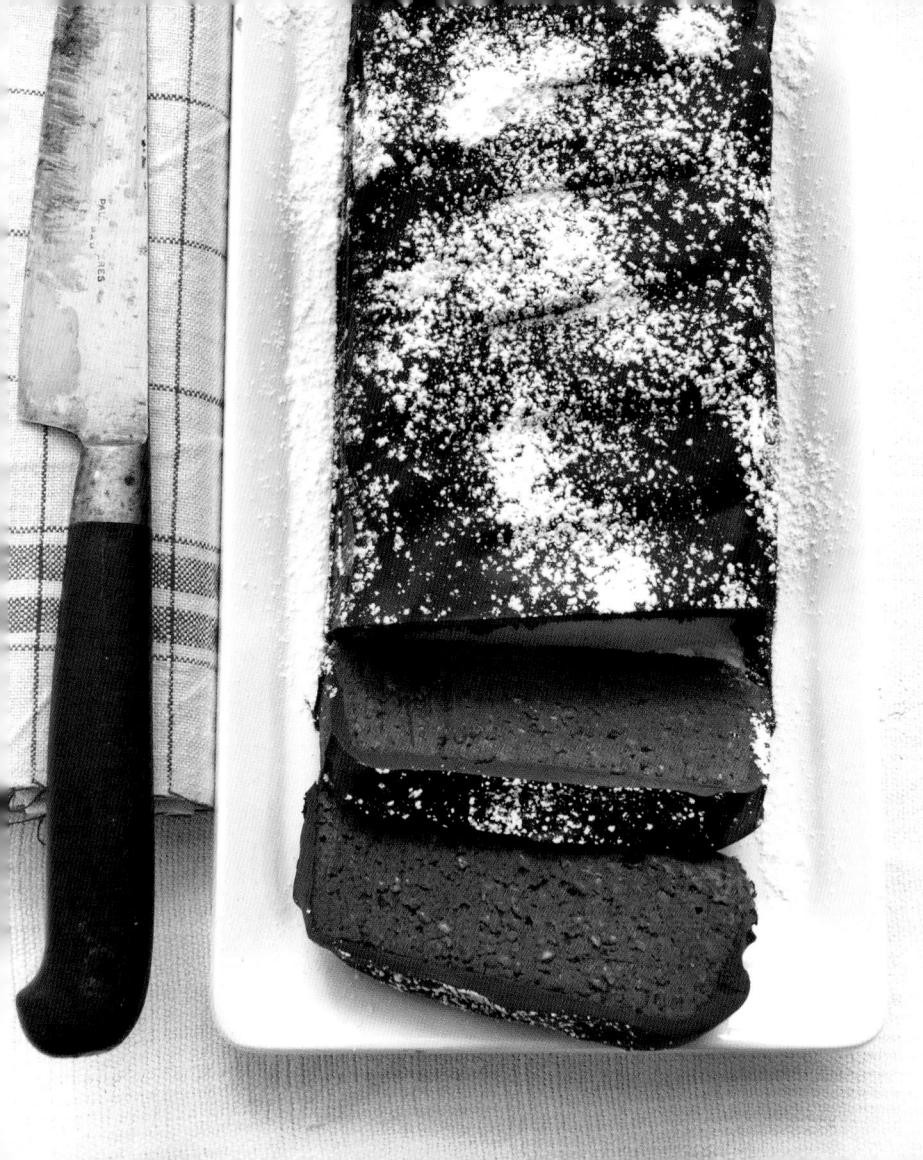

Double ginger gingerbread men

Even the smallest hands can help make these friendly little fellows. Box them up and tie with a pretty ribbon to make a lovely gift for someone special at Christmas.

TAKES 1 HOUR ● MAKES 12 BIG GINGERBREAD MEN

140g/5oz unsalted butter
100g/4oz dark muscovado sugar
3 tbsp golden syrup
175g/6oz buckwheat flour
175g/6oz gluten-free plain flour
1 tsp bicarbonate of soda
2 tsp ground ginger
1 tsp ground cinnamon
pinch cayenne pepper (optional)
2 balls stem ginger from a jar, chopped

TO DECORATE

50g/2oz icing sugar
a few glacé cherries
2 balls stem ginger

1 Heat oven to 200C/180C fan/gas 6. Line two baking sheets with parchment. Melt the butter, sugar and syrup in a pan. Mix the flours, bicarb, spices and a pinch of salt in a bowl. Stir in the butter mix and stem ginger to make a stiff-ish dough.

2 Wait until it is cool enough to handle, then roll out the dough to about 5mm/¼in thick. Stamp out 12 gingerbread men, re-rolling and pressing the trimmings back together and rolling again. Lift on to the baking sheets. Bake for 12 minutes until golden. Cool for 10 minutes on the sheets, then lift on to cooling racks.

3 To decorate, mix icing sugar with a few drops of water until thick and smooth. Halve then slice the cherries thinly to make smiles, and cut the ginger into small squares. Spoon the icing into a food bag, snip off the tiniest bit from one corner, then squeeze eyes and buttons and a smile on to one man at a time. Stick on a cherry smile and ginger buttons. Repeat; leave to set.

PER BISCUIT 264 kcals, protein 3g, carbs 43g, fat 10g, sat fat 6g, fibre 1g, sugar 20g, salt 0.33g

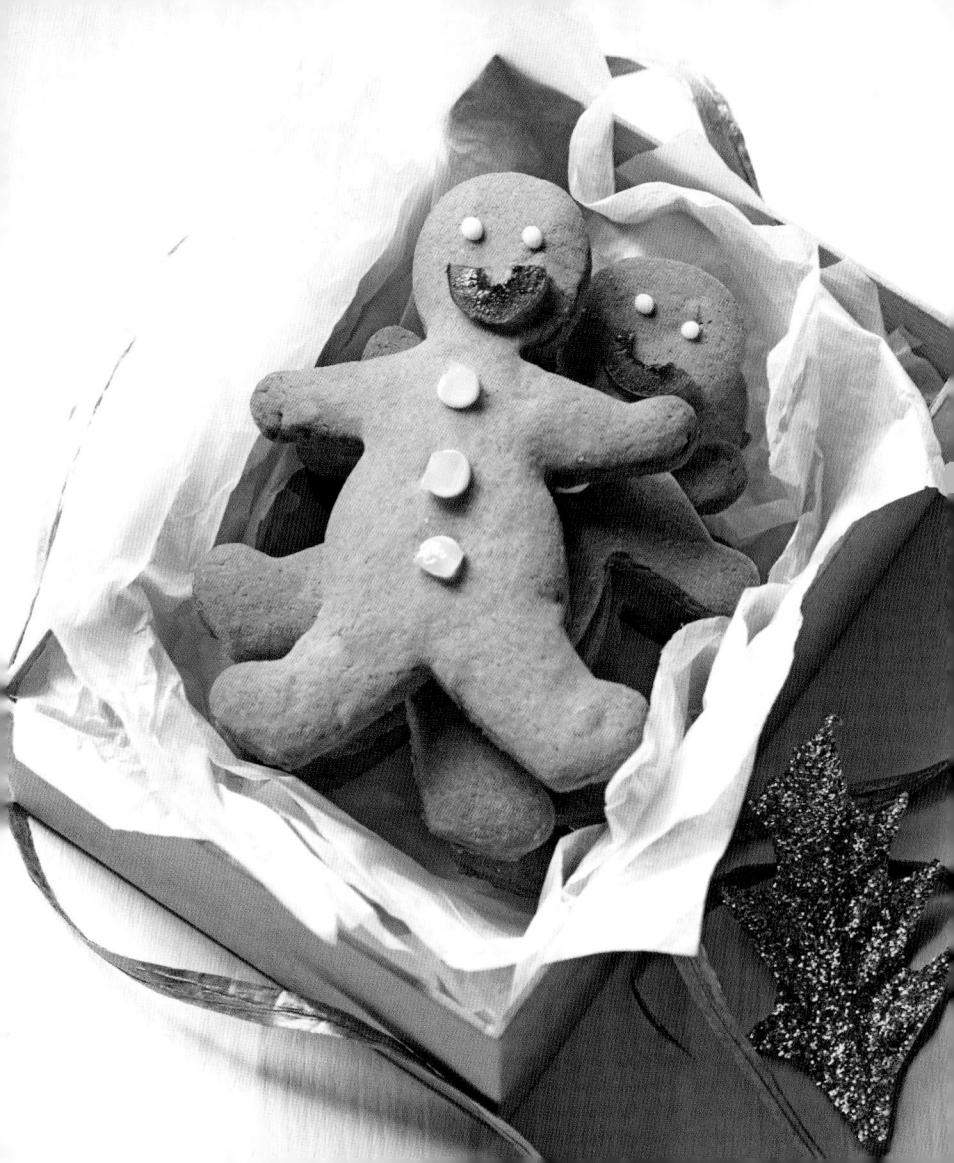

Cappuccino cake

A traybake is one of the easiest cakes to make and portion up afterward; so it's ideal for coffee mornings, birthday teas or charity cake sales.

TAKES 50 MINUTES • CUTS INTO 15 SQUARES

250g/9oz softened butter, plus extra for greasing

200g/7oz gluten-free self-raising flour (add 2 tsp xanthan gum, if it doesn't contain any)

100g/4oz ground almonds

250g/9oz golden caster sugar

1 tsp gluten-free baking powder

4 large eggs

150g pot natural yogurt

1 tsp vanilla paste or extract

1 tbsp cocoa powder, plus extra to dust

100ml/3½fl oz strong coffee (use 2 tbsp coffee granules)

140g/5oz icing sugar, sifted

350g/12oz mascarpone or soft cheese

few chocolate-covered coffee beans, to scatter

1 Heat oven to 180C/160C fan/gas 4. Grease a 20 × 30cm baking or roasting tin and line with baking parchment. Beat the butter, flour, almonds, sugar, baking powder, eggs, yogurt, vanilla, cocoa and half the coffee in a large bowl with an electric whisk until lump-free. Spoon into the tin, then bake for 25–30 minutes until golden and risen, and a skewer poked in comes out clean. Drizzle with the remaining coffee.

2 Cool in the tin while you stir the icing sugar into the mascarpone or soft cheese. Spread the icing over the cooled cake, dust with a little cocoa and scatter with the coffee beans.

PER SQUARE 436 kcals, protein 5g, carbs 45g, fat 28g, sat fat 16g, fibre 1g, sugar 31g, salt 0.56g

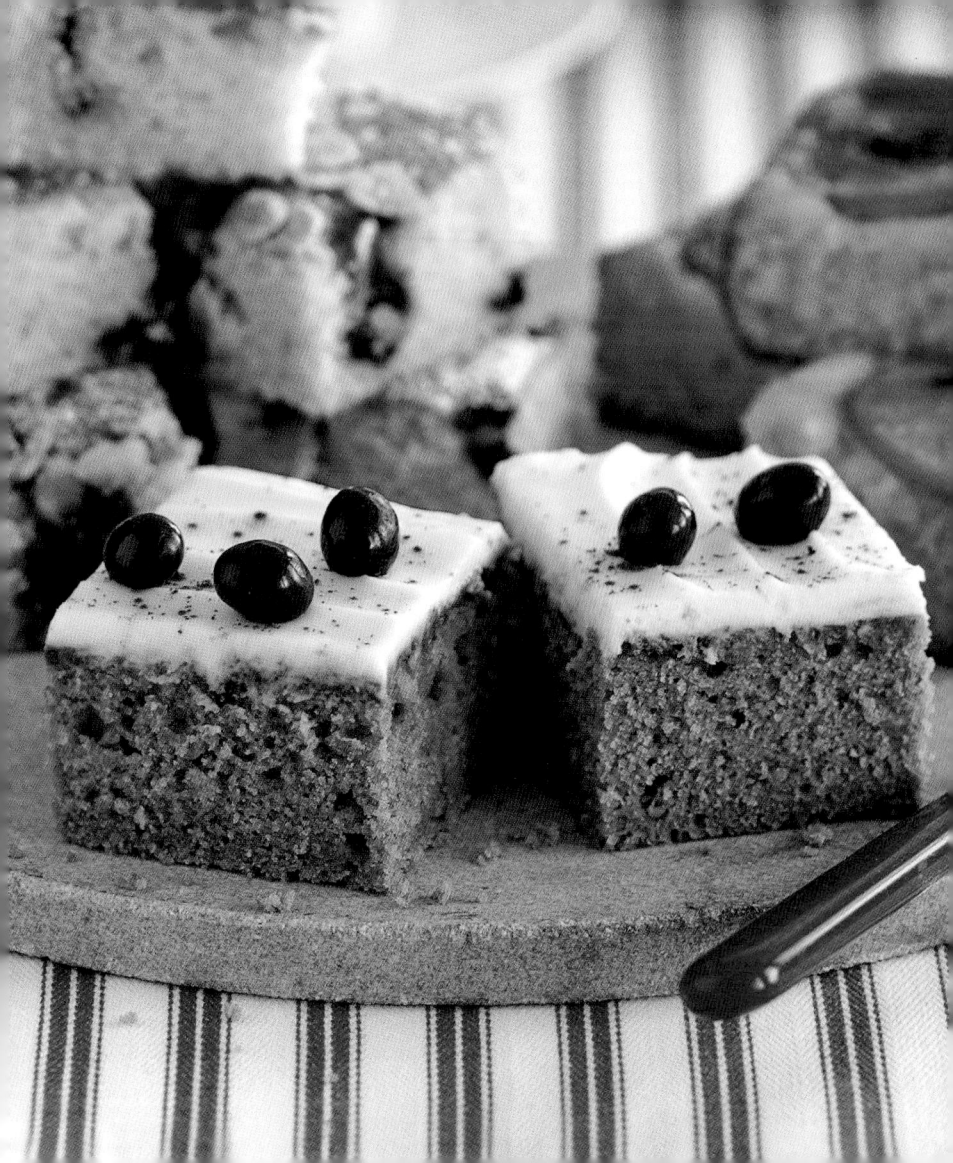

Summer fruit bowl tartlets

These make a cute addition to an afternoon tea for the girls, or serve as a smart dessert at a dinner party.

TAKES 45 MINUTES, PLUS COOLING
● **MAKES 8**

300ml/½ pint milk
1 tsp vanilla paste
3 large egg yolks
50g/2oz caster sugar
1 rounded tbsp cornflour
knob of butter
400g/14oz mixed summer berries, or
    strawberries halved or quartered
icing sugar and a few chopped
    pistachios, to decorate (optional)

FOR THE PASTRY
120g/4½oz chilled butter, diced
200g/7oz gluten-free plain flour, plus
    a little extra for dusting
1 tbsp icing sugar

1 To make the pastry, rub butter into the flour to fine breadcrumbs. Stir in the icing sugar. Add 4 tablespoons water, mixing with a cutlery knife until the dough starts to come together. Knead lightly, wrap in cling film and chill for at least 30 minutes.

2 Heat the milk until just steaming. Whisk the vanilla, egg yolks, sugar and cornflour. Keep whisking while pouring in the milk. Bring slowly to the boil in a pan, stirring, until the custard is thickened and smooth – beating out the lumps as it cooks. Cool.

3 Heat oven to 190C/170C fan/gas 5. Divide the pastry into eight and roll out each to line a 7–8cm deep tartlet tin. Line each with a paper cake case and some baking beans. Bake for 10 minutes, then remove the paper and beans and bake for a further 5 minutes until the pastry is golden. Remove from the tins and cool on a wire rack.

4 Fill with cooled custard and pile on fruits. Dust with icing sugar and scatter over chopped pistachios, if you like.

PER SERVING 281 kcals, protein 5g, carbs 32g, fat 15g, sat fat 6g, fibre 2g, sugar 14g, salt 0.46g

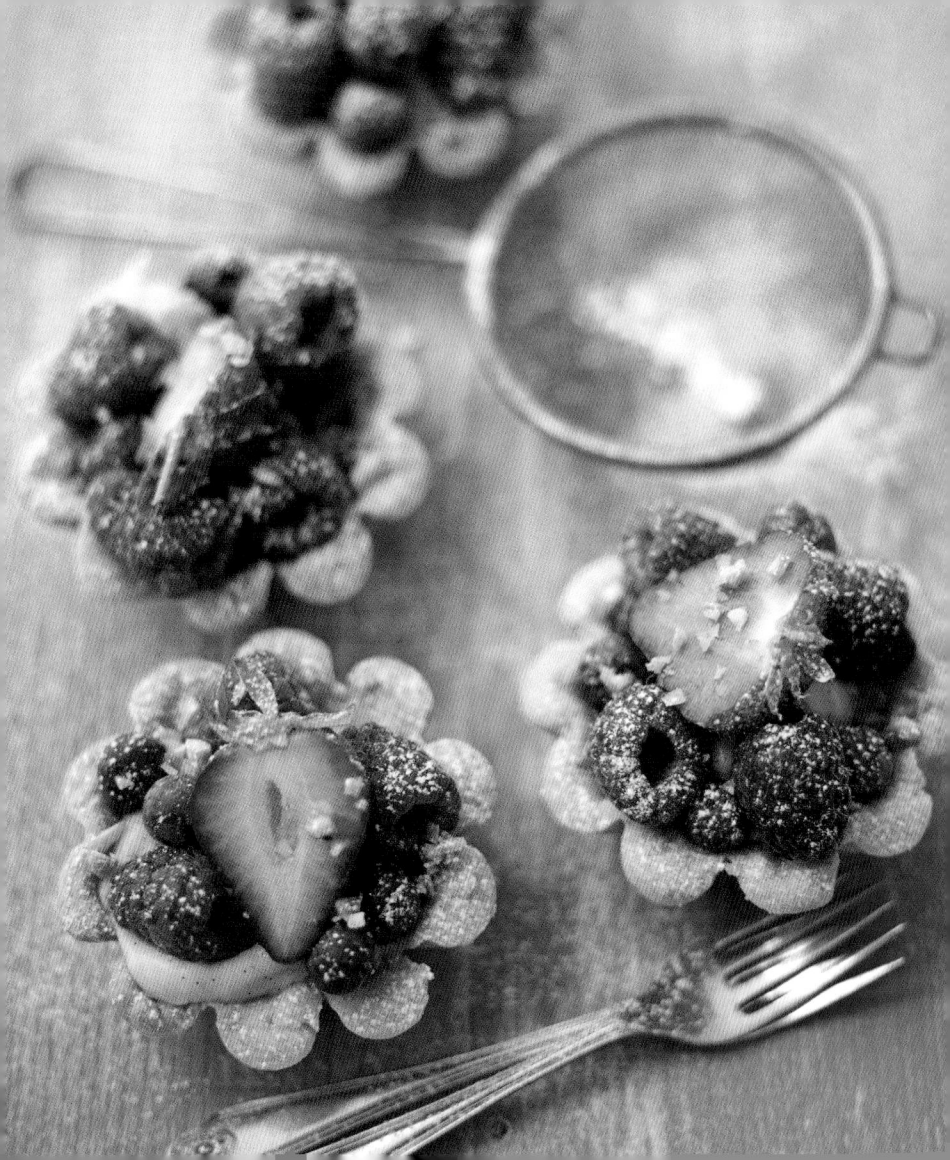

Self-saucing Jaffa pudding

This pud starts life as an ugly duckling, but don't fear as the hot watery sauce floats among the batter – once you bake it, you'll end up with something beautiful.

TAKES 1 HOUR 10 MINUTES

● **SERVES 8**

100g/4oz butter, melted, plus a little extra for the dish
200g/7oz gluten-free plain flour
50g/2oz buckwheat flour
140g/5oz caster sugar
50g/2oz cocoa powder
1 tbsp gluten-free baking powder
2 tsp xanthan gum
zest and juice 1 orange
3 large eggs
150ml/¼ pint milk
100g/4oz orange milk chocolate or milk chocolate, broken into chunks
vanilla ice cream or single cream, to serve

FOR THE SAUCE

200g/7oz light muscovado sugar
25g/1oz cocoa powder

1 Butter a 2-litre, not too deep, baking dish and heat oven to 180C/160C fan/gas 4. Put the kettle on. Put the flours, caster sugar, cocoa, baking powder, xanthan gum, orange zest and a pinch of salt in a large mixing bowl. Whisk together the orange juice and any pulp left in the juicer, the eggs, melted butter and milk, then pour on to the dry ingredients and mix together until smooth. Stir in the chocolate chunks and scrape everything into the baking dish.

2 Mix 300ml/½ pint boiling water from the kettle with the sugar and cocoa for the sauce, then pour this all over the pudding batter – don't worry, it will look very strange at this stage! Bake on the middle shelf of the oven for 30 minutes until the surface looks firm, risen and crisp. As you scoop spoonfuls into serving bowls, you should find a glossy, rich chocolate sauce underneath the sponge. Eat immediately with vanilla ice cream or single cream.

PER SERVING 522 kcals, protein 8g, carbs 82g, fat 21g, sat fat 11g, fibre 2g, sugar 54g, salt 0.86g

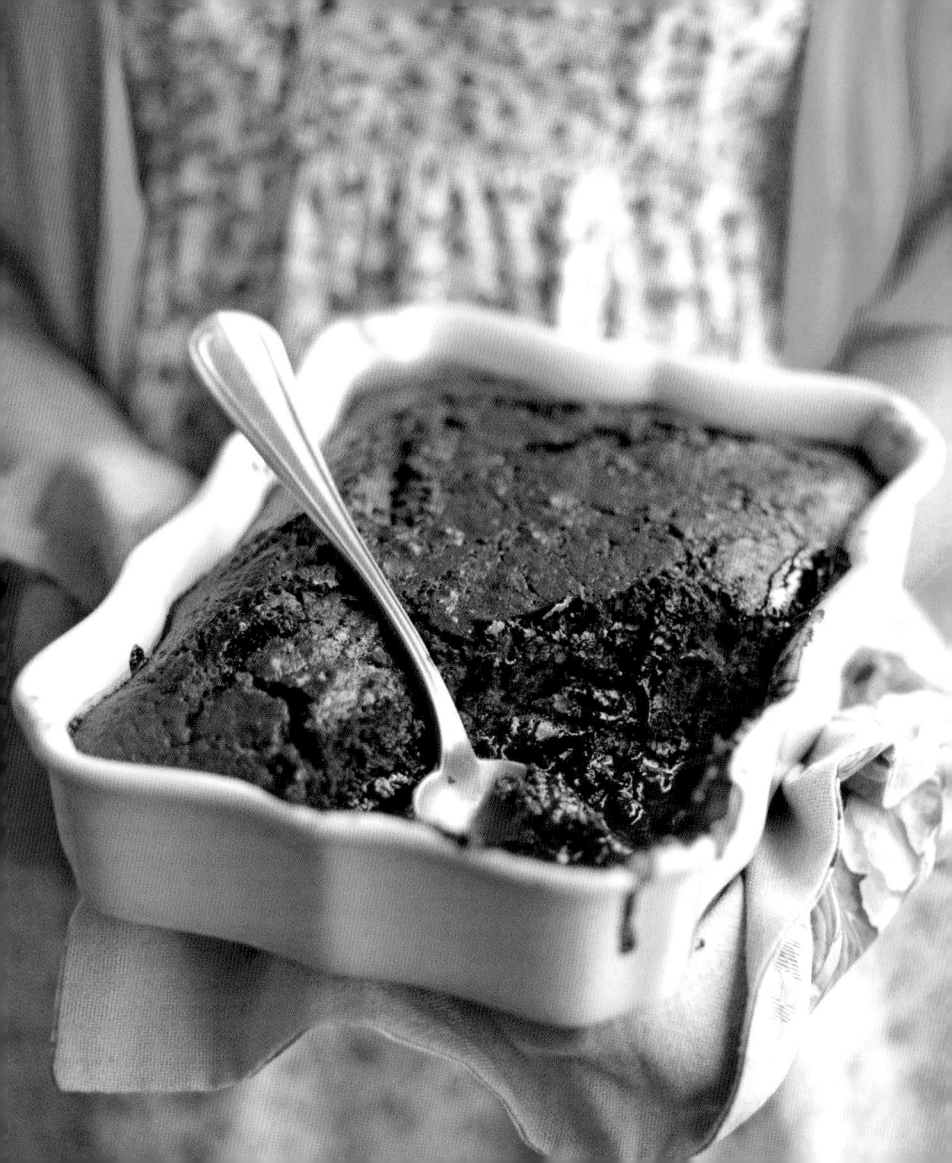

Berry slump

This cleverly uses frozen summer berries; so it makes a great fruity pudding any time of the year. Serve it up after Sunday lunch and you'll put a smile on everyone's face.

TAKES 40 MINUTES ● SERVES 4–6

100g/4oz butter, softened, plus extra
  for greasing
100g/4oz caster sugar, plus extra
  2 tbsp
100g/4oz gluten-free flour
1 tsp each gluten-free baking powder
  and xanthan gum
2 eggs
1 tbsp milk
2 tsp vanilla extract
600g/1lb 5oz frozen mixed summer
  berries
25g/1oz flaked almonds
custard or vanilla ice cream, to serve

1 Heat oven to 180C/160C fan/gas 4. In a food processor, whizz together the butter, sugar, flour, baking powder, xanthan gum, eggs, milk and 1 teaspoon of the vanilla extract until smooth. Lightly grease a roughly oval 20 × 30cm baking dish, then tip in the frozen fruit. Scatter over the extra sugar and remaining vanilla extract. Dollop the cake mix over the sugar and fruit, then smooth all over with the back of a spoon to cover the fruit. Make a little dip in the middle of the mixture to ensure it cooks evenly throughout. Scatter over the almonds.
2 Cook for 45 minutes until the fruit is hot and the sponge is cooked through. Serve warm with custard or vanilla ice cream.

PER SERVING (4) 530 kcals, protein 9g, carbs 64g, fat 28g, sat fat 14g, fibre 5g, sugar 46g, salt 0.78g

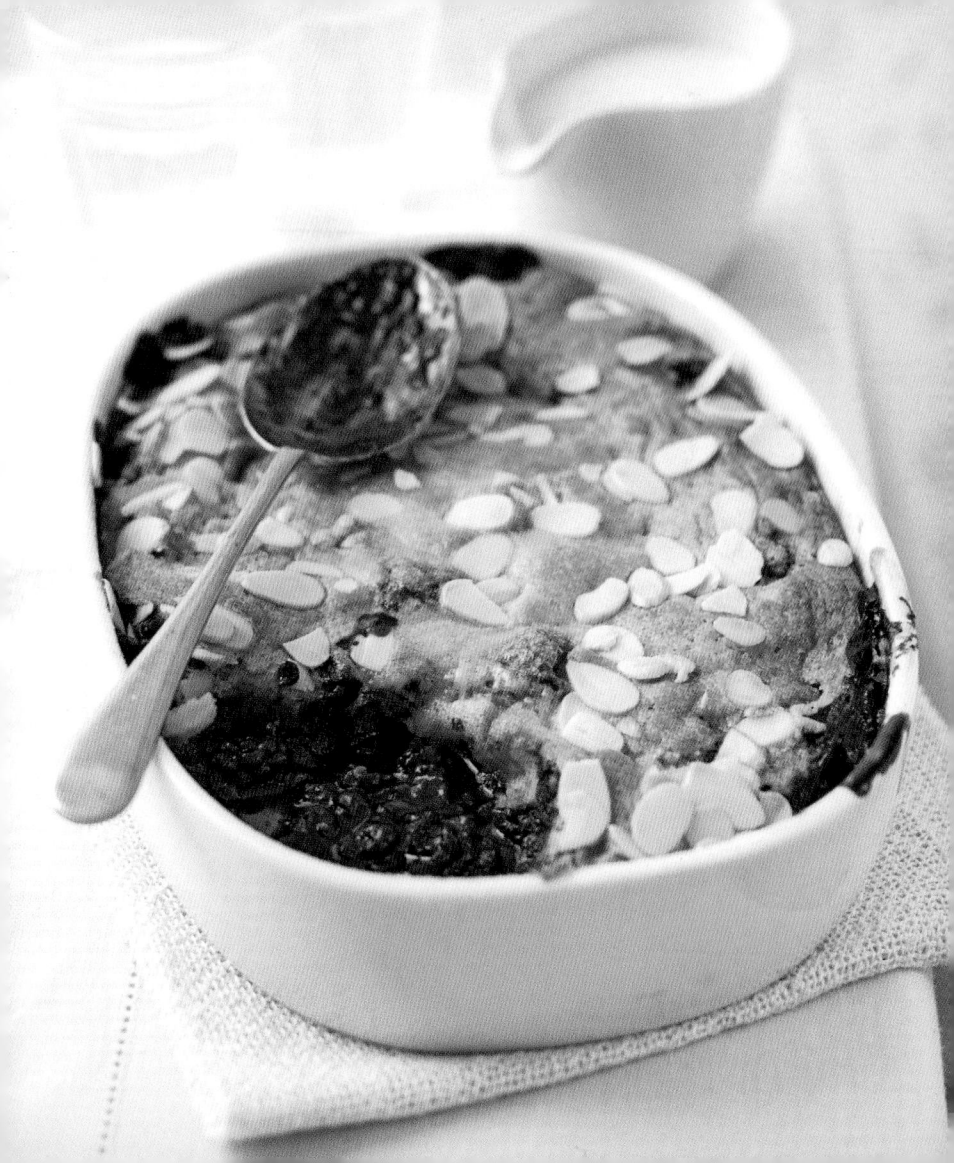

Chocolate–courgette cake

You can use one overgrown courgette here, but peel first and take out the seeds. As courgettes vary so much in size, you measure them by volume in this clever recipe.

TAKES 1 HOUR 10 MINUTES, PLUS COOLING • SERVES 10

250g/9oz gluten-free plain flour
100g/4oz ground almonds
2 tsp each baking powder and xanthan gum
50g/2oz cocoa powder
1 tsp mixed spice
175ml/6fl oz extra virgin olive oil
375g/13oz golden caster sugar
3 large eggs
2 tsp vanilla essence
500ml/18fl oz grated courgette (measure by volume in a measuring jug)
140g/5oz toasted hazelnuts, roughly chopped

FOR THE ICING

200g/7oz dark chocolate, chopped
100ml/3½fl oz double cream

1 Heat oven to 180C/160C fan/gas 4 and line a 24cm cake tin with baking parchment. In a large bowl, combine the flour, almonds, baking powder and xanthan gum, cocoa powder, mixed spice and 1 teaspoon salt. In another bowl, combine the olive oil, sugar, eggs, vanilla essence and grated courgette. Mix the dry and wet mixtures until just combined, then fold in the toasted hazelnuts and scrape into the tin. Bake for about 40–50 minutes, or until a knife inserted into the middle comes out clean. Cool in the tin for 10 minutes, then turn out on to a wire rack and leave to cool.

2 To make the icing, put the chocolate in a bowl and bring the cream to the boil in a pan. Pour the hot cream over the chocolate and stir until melted. Cool to thicken slightly, then spread over the cake.

PER SERVING 716 kcals, protein 10g, carbs 84g, fat 40g, sat fat 10g, fibre 4g, sugar 55g, salt 0.43g

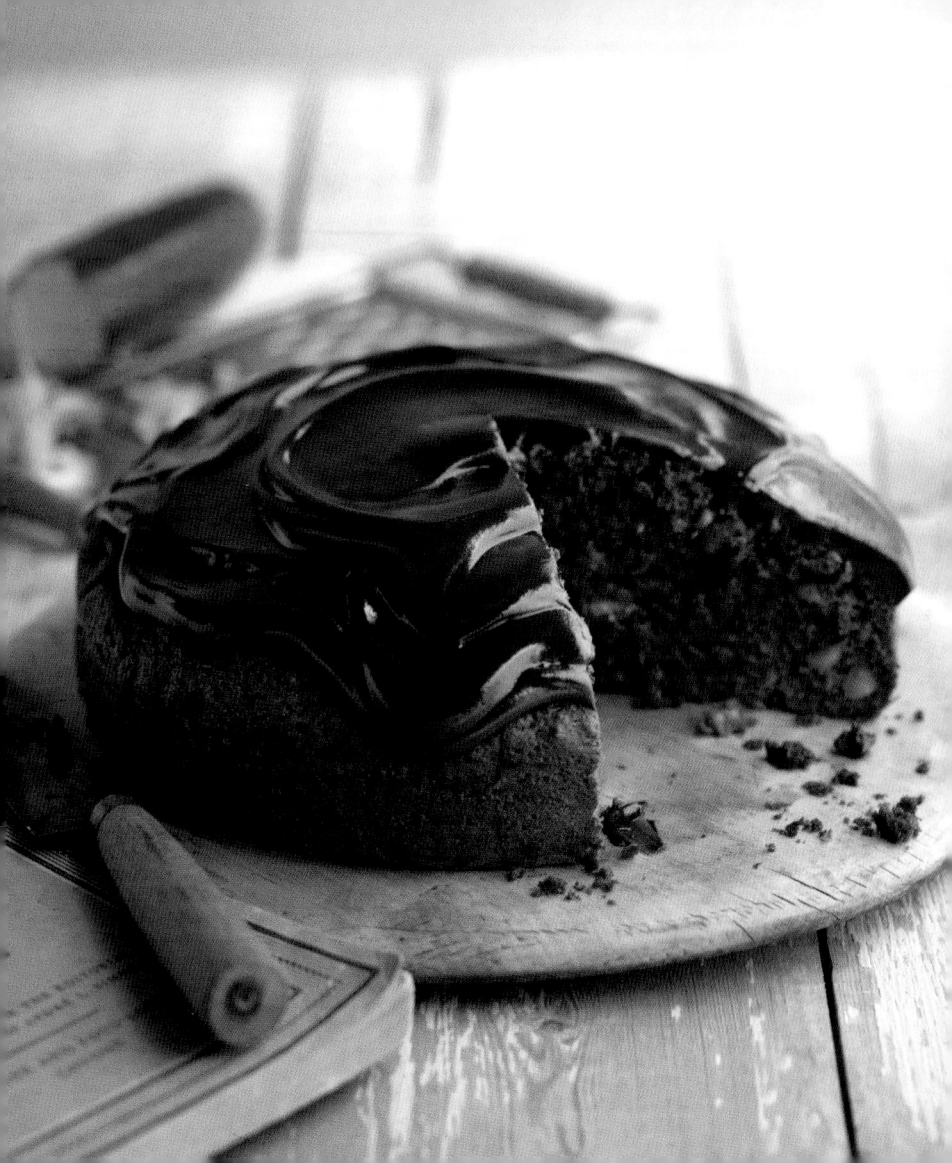

Frozen banana & peanut butter cheesecake

Once made, this is a great standby that can be pulled out at a moment's notice. The combination of banana and peanut butter will impress children and adults alike.

TAKES 30 MINUTES, PLUS FREEZING

● **SERVES 8–10**

3 small bananas
50g/2oz butter, melted
10 gluten-free digestive biscuits, crushed to crumbs
150ml tub double cream
140g/5oz icing sugar
400g tub soft cheese
½ tsp vanilla extract
237g jar gluten-free crunchy peanut butter

1 Several hours before, put 2 of the bananas in the freezer until the skins go black, then remove and defrost. You'll be left with really soft bananas. Peel, then mash well and set aside.

2 Mix the butter and biscuits together, then press into a 22cm-round springform cake tin. Whip the cream until it just holds its shape. In a separate bowl, beat the sugar, soft cheese and vanilla together until completely combined. In another bowl, beat the peanut butter to loosen it.

3 Fold the cheese mixture into the peanut butter, then tip in the mashed banana and gently fold in the cream. Spread the mix over the biscuit base and smooth the top. Freeze for several hours or preferably overnight. To serve, leave the cheesecake in the fridge for 20 minutes, then run a knife around the edge and remove the sides of the tin. Slice the remaining banana and use to decorate the cheesecake.

PER SERVING (8) 624 kcals, protein 12g, carbs 43g, fat 46g, sat fat 21g, fibre 3g, sugar 30g, salt 1.18g

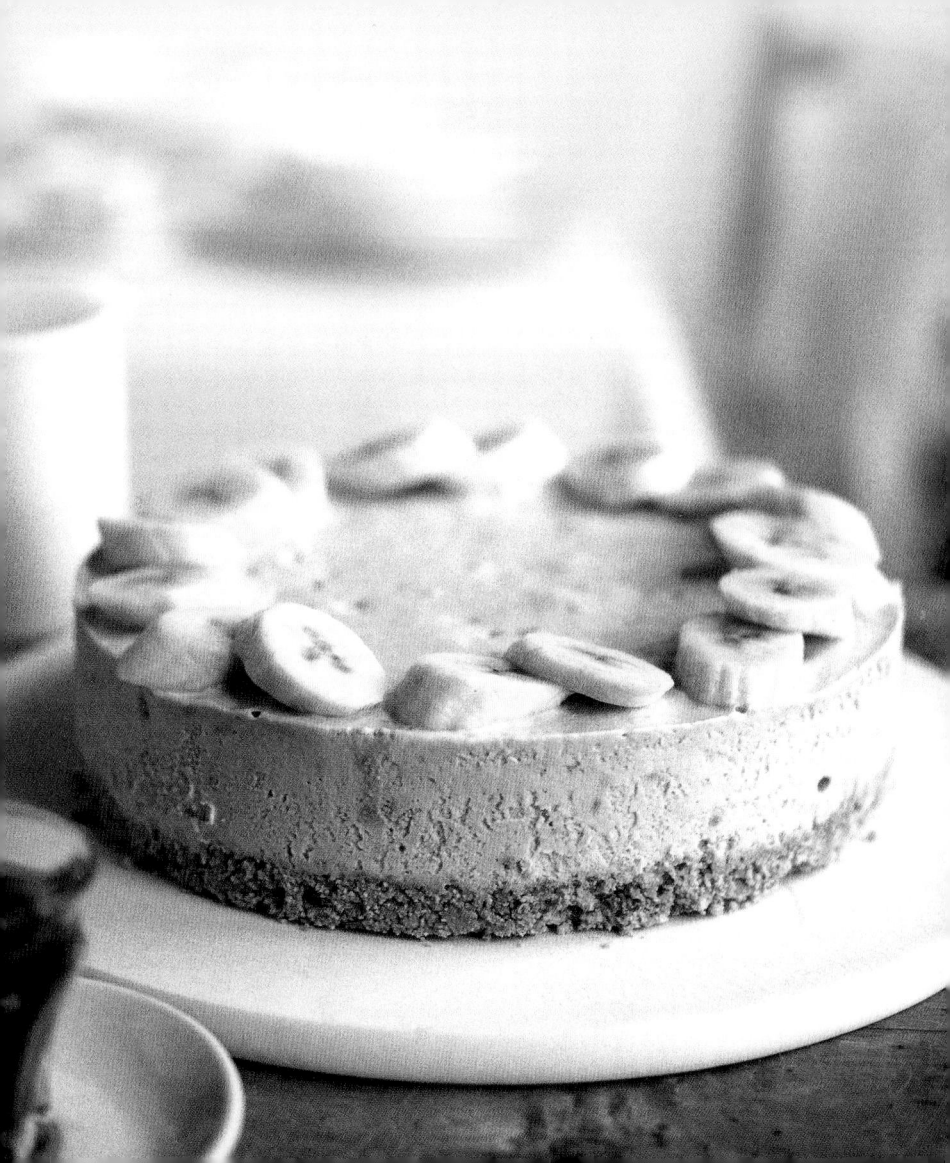

Hazelnut meringue surprise

This layered meringue cake would work just as well for pudding as it would for a special afternoon tea.

TAKES 55 MINUTES • SERVES 8

a little butter, for greasing
200g/7oz hazelnuts
25g/1oz icing sugar
6 egg whites
450g/1lb golden caster sugar
1 tsp vanilla extract
1 tsp cornflour
200g/7oz dark chocolate, chopped
400ml/14fl oz double cream
200g/7oz raspberries

1 Heat oven to 190C/170C fan/gas 5. Butter and line the bases and sides of two 20cm-round springform tins with baking parchment. Whizz the hazelnuts and icing sugar in a food processor until fine.
2 Whisk the egg whites until stiff, add half the caster sugar and whisk again, then repeat with the rest of the caster sugar. Fold in the vanilla, cornflour and ground nut mixture. Divide the mixture between the tins and bake for 25–30 minutes until the tops are firm. Remove and cool.
3 Meanwhile, make the chocolate cream. Melt the chocolate in a bowl over a pan of barely simmering water, then remove from the heat. Leave to cool slightly, then stir in the cream and leave to set in a cool place.
4 Remove the meringues from the tins. Crush half of the berries. Spread half the chocolate cream over one meringue and spoon over the crushed berries. Top with the second meringue, then ice with chocolate cream and decorate with the remaining berries. Chill until serving.

PER SERVING 764 kcals, protein 9g, carbs 83g, fat 47g, sat fat 20g, fibre 3g, sugar 82g, salt 0.18g

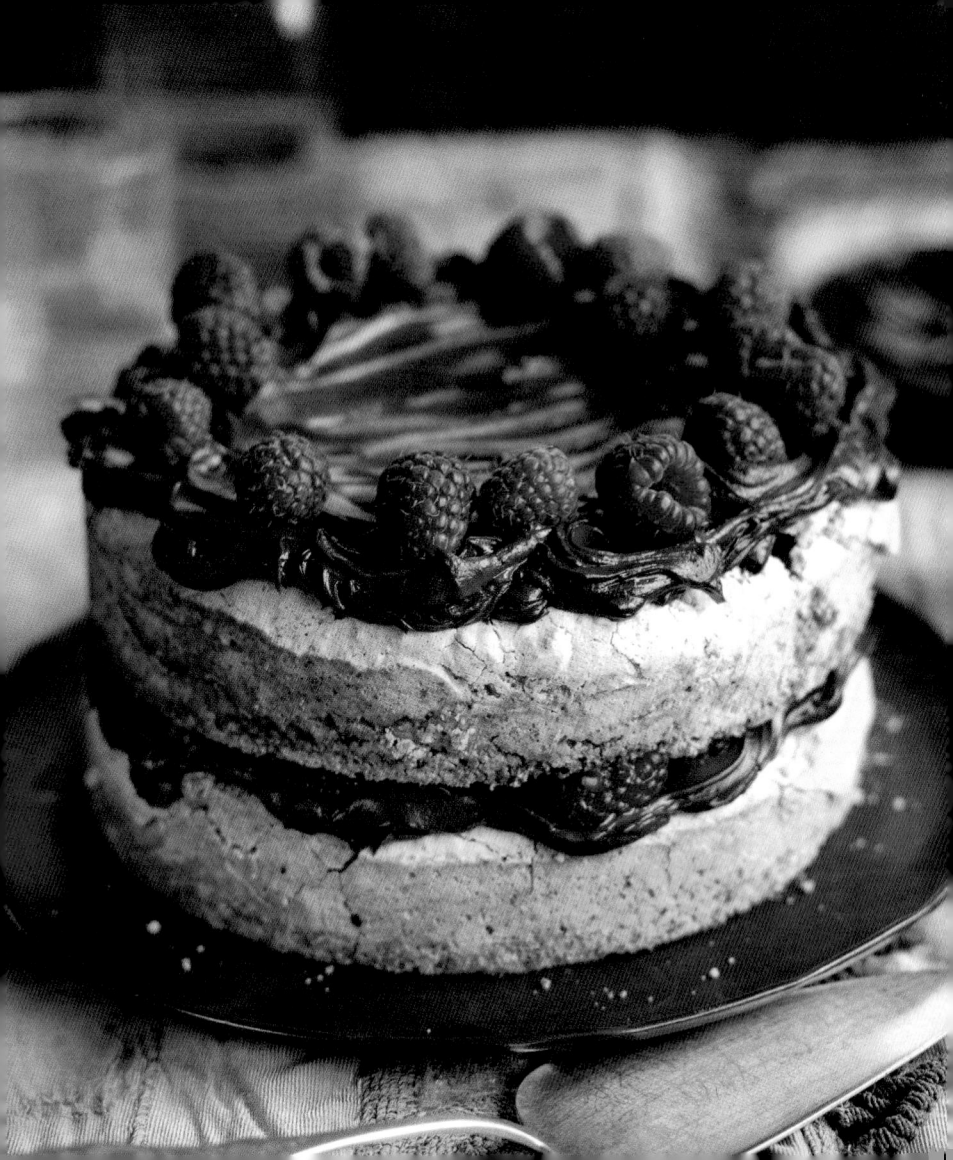

Cherry shortbread hearts

Why not box up these biscuits as a gift for someone you love on Valentine's Day?
(Or just treat yourself with a cup of tea!)

TAKES 30 MINUTES ● MAKES 14–16, DEPENDING ON CUTTER

100g/4oz icing sugar, plus extra for dusting
100g/4oz gluten-free plain flour, plus extra for rolling
100g/4oz rice flour
50g/2oz cornflour
50g/2oz ground almonds
250g pack cold butter, cut into cubes
50g/2oz glacé cherries, finely chopped
½ tsp almond extract
8 tbsp cherry jam, sieved

1 Heat oven to 180C/160C fan/gas 4. Sift the icing sugar, flours and cornflour together into a bowl. Stir in the ground almonds and butter, then rub in the butter until smooth. Stir in the chopped glacé cherries and almond extract, and bring together to form a dough.
2 Roll out on a lightly floured surface, then stamp out biscuits using a heart-shaped cutter. Keep re-rolling the trimmings until all the dough is used. Carefully transfer the biscuits to baking sheets lined with parchment and bake for 8–10 minutes until just pale golden.
3 Using an upturned bottle top or similar, press gently into the centre of each biscuit to make a round indent. Spoon in a little jam and return to the oven for 2 minutes. Remove and cool on a wire rack, before dusting with icing sugar to serve.

PER SERVING (16) 242 kcals, protein 2g, carbs 27g, fat 15g, sat fat 8g, fibre 1g, sugar 14g, salt 0.21g

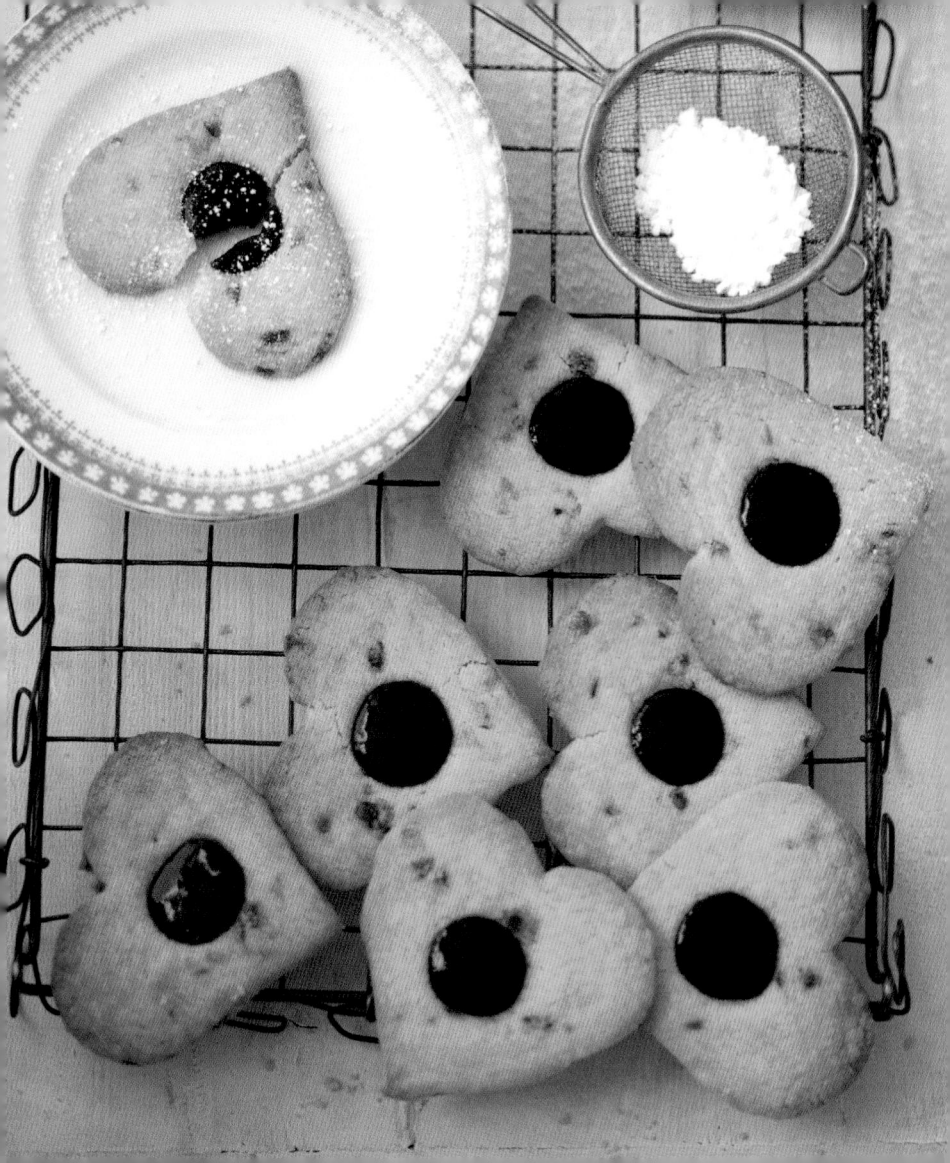

Banana, walnut & chocolate chip loaf

Whip up one of the easiest bakes ever and enjoy warm from the oven for breakfast, morning or afternoon tea – in fact any excuse at all!

TAKES 1 HOUR 20 MINUTES

- **SERVES 8**

4 ripe bananas, peeled

250g/9oz caster sugar

2 large eggs

140g/5oz softened butter

250g/9oz gluten-free plain flour

1 tsp each gluten-free baking powder and xanthan gum

100g/4oz walnut pieces, roughly chopped

100g/4oz chocolate chips

1 Heat oven to 190C/170C fan/gas 5. Line a 900g loaf tin with baking parchment. In a large bowl, mash together the bananas and the sugar with the back of a fork. Add the eggs and mix well with an electric hand whisk until fully incorporated, then add the butter and mix for a couple of minutes more to blend everything together. Sieve in the flour, baking powder and xanthan gum, and fold together with a spatula, then add the walnuts and chocolate chips. Give everything one final mix before tipping into the lined loaf tin.

2 Bake for 1 hour 5 minutes or until a skewer inserted into the middle comes out clean. Leave to cool slightly in the tin, then turn out and serve cut into thick slices, either warm or at room temperature.

PER SERVING 578 kcals, protein 8g, carbs 72g, fat 28g, sat fat 13g, fibre 2g, sugar 50g, salt 0.6g

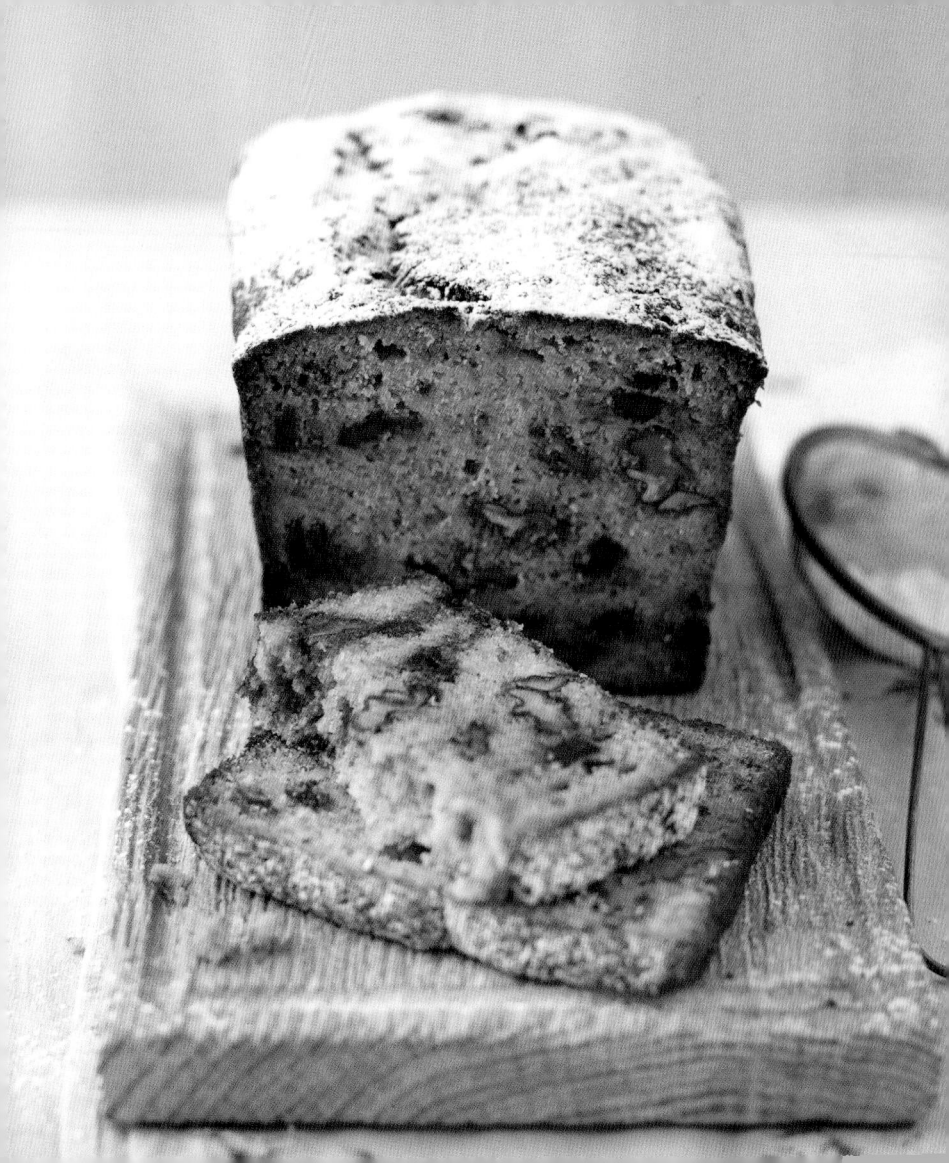

Chocolate & raspberry brownies

These are possibly the best brownies you'll ever taste, and super-super gooey. If you fancy them a little firmer, just bake them for a few more minutes.

TAKES 50 MINUTES • CUTS INTO 15 SQUARES

200g/7oz dark chocolate, broken into chunks

100g/4oz milk chocolate, broken into chunks

250g pack salted butter

400g/14oz light soft brown sugar

4 large eggs

140g/5oz gluten-free plain flour

50g/2oz cocoa powder

200g/7oz raspberries

1 Heat oven to 180C/160C fan/gas 4. Line a 20 × 30cm baking tin with baking parchment. Put the chocolate, butter and sugar in a pan and gently melt, stirring occasionally with a wooden spoon. Remove from the heat.

2 Stir the eggs, one by one, into the melted-chocolate mixture, sieve over the flour and cocoa, and stir in. Stir in half the raspberries, scrape into the tin, then scatter over the remaining raspberries. Bake on the middle shelf for 30 minutes or, if you prefer a firmer texture, for 5 minutes more. Cool before slicing into squares. Store in an airtight container for up to 3 days.

PER SERVING 389 kcals, protein 5g, carbs 44g, fat 22g, sat fat 13g, fibre 2g, sugar 38g, salt 0.4g

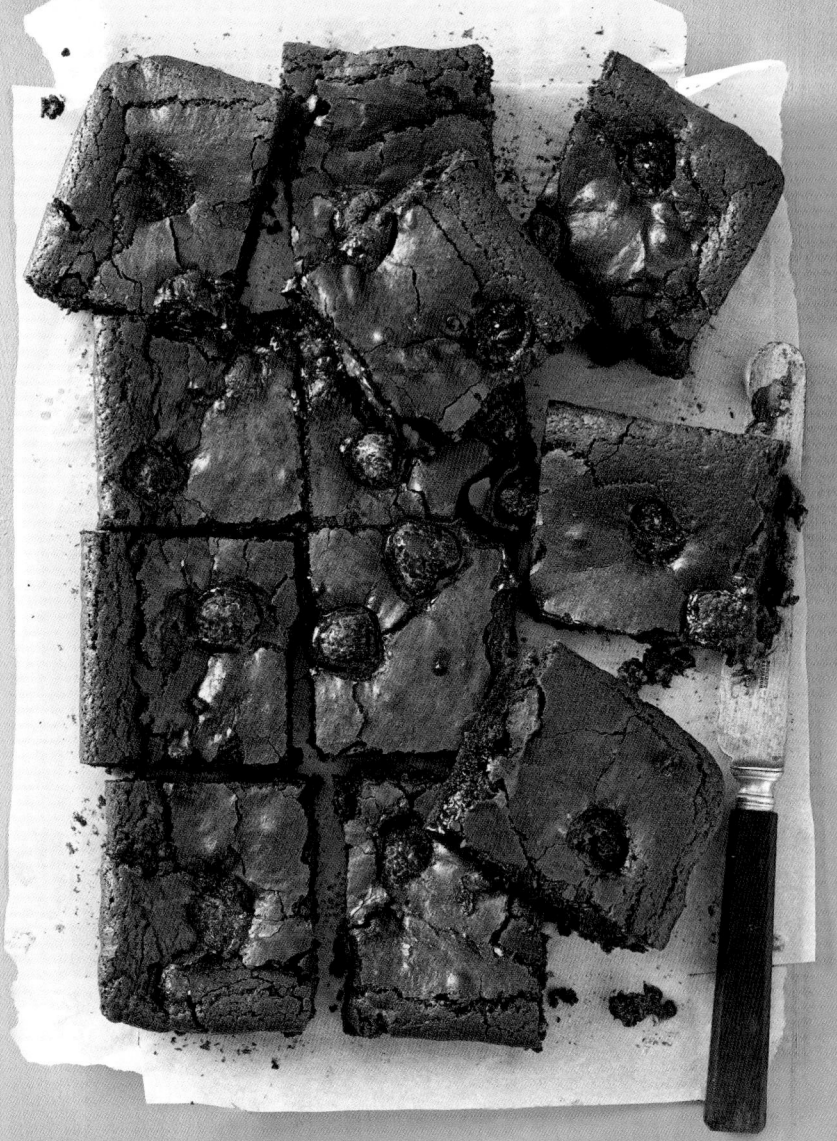

Lighter lemon drizzle cake

This recipe gives a smooth, syrupy lemon topping that soaks into the cake.

TAKES 1 HOUR 10 MINUTES

● **CUTS INTO 12 SLICES**

75ml/2½fl oz rapeseed oil, plus extra
  for the tin
175g/6oz gluten-free self-raising flour
  (add 2 tsp xanthan gum, if it doesn't
  contain any)
1½ tsp gluten-free baking powder
50g/2oz each ground almonds and
  polenta
zest 2 lemons
140g/5oz golden caster sugar
2 large eggs
225g/8oz natural yogurt

FOR THE LEMON SYRUP

85g/3oz caster sugar
juice 2 lemons (about 5 tbsp)

1 Heat oven to 180C/160C fan/gas 4. Grease a deep 20cm-round cake tin and line the base with baking parchment. Put the flour, baking powder, ground almonds, polenta, lemon zest and sugar in a bowl. Beat the eggs and the yogurt, and tip into the dry ingredients with the oil. Fold together without over-mixing.

2 Spoon into the tin and bake for 40 minutes. Cover loosely with foil for the final 5–10 minutes if it browns too quickly.

3 Meanwhile, make the syrup. Tip the sugar and lemon juice into a pan with 75ml/2½fl oz water. Heat, stirring occasionally, until the sugar has dissolved. Raise the heat, boil for 4 minutes until slightly reduced, then remove from the heat.

4 Cool the cake for 15 minutes in the tin, then remove it from the tin and sit it on a wire rack set over a baking tin. Poke lots of holes over the surface using a skewer and gradually spoon over the syrup, letting it soak in between additions.

PER SLICE 243 kcals, protein 5g, carbs 35g, fat 10g, sat fat 1.4g, fibre 0.9g, sugar 22g, salt 0.34g

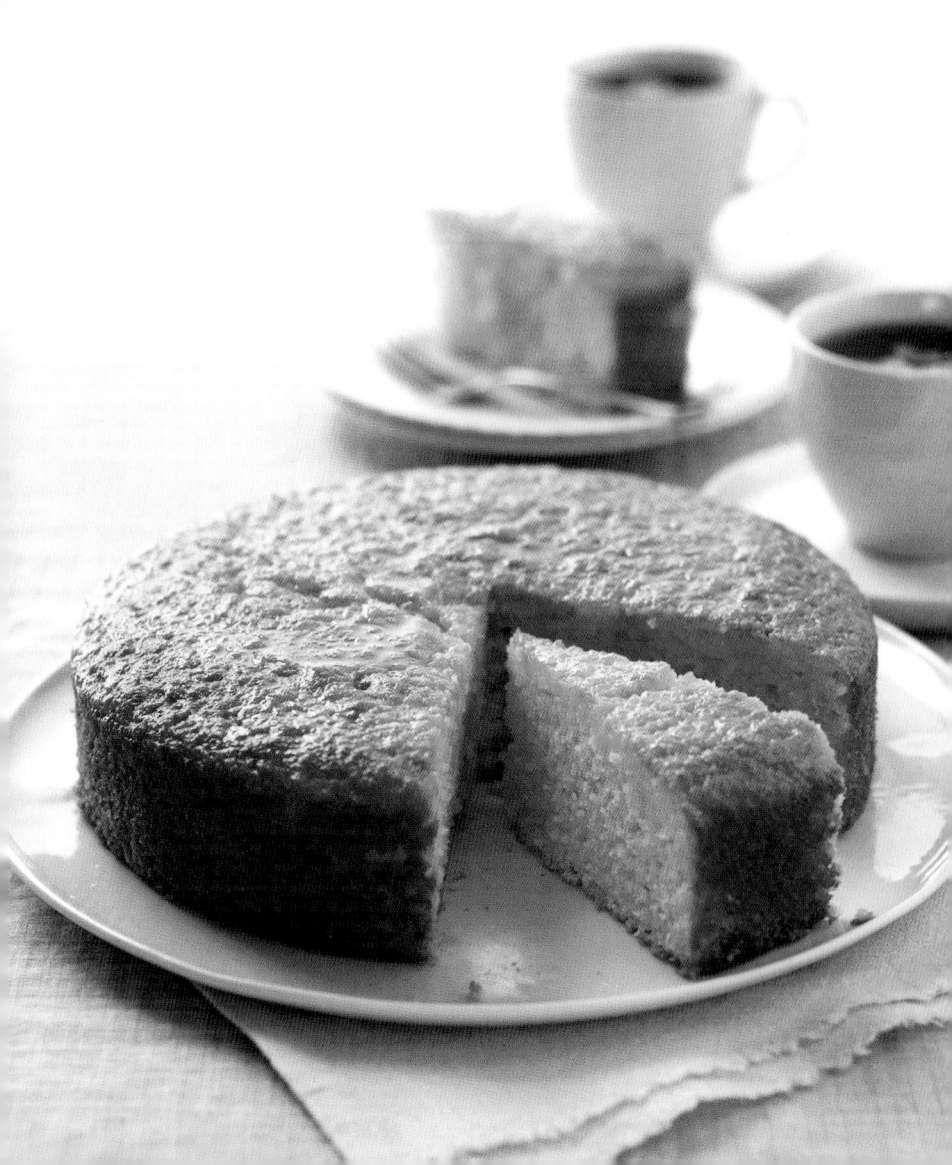

Chocolate & pecan tart

This make-ahead pud will become a real family favourite – a cross between pecan pie and chocolate tart, what's not to love?

TAKES 1¾ HOURS • SERVES 6–8

175g/6oz dark chocolate
50g/2oz salted butter
4 eggs, beaten
250ml/9fl oz maple syrup
250g/9oz whole pecan nuts
vanilla ice cream or double cream,
    to serve

FOR THE PASTRY

150g/5½oz cold butter, diced
250g/9oz gluten-free plain flour, plus
    extra for rolling
1½ tsp xanthan gum
2 tbsp icing sugar

1 To make the pastry, rub the butter into the flour until the mixture resembles fine breadcrumbs. Stir in the xanthan gum and icing sugar. Add 5 tablespoons water, mixing with a cutlery knife until the dough starts to come together. Knead lightly, wrap in cling film and chill for at least 30 minutes.

2 Heat oven to 180C/160C fan/gas 4. Roll the pastry out on a lightly floured surface and use to line a 20cm-round loose-bottomed tart tin. Fill the tart with baking paper and baking beans, bake for 25 minutes, then remove the paper and beans. Continue to cook for 10 minutes until golden. Remove from the oven; cool.

3 Melt the chocolate and butter together in a large bowl over a pan of simmering water. Whisk the eggs and maple syrup together, then stir into the chocolate with most of the nuts. Pour into the tart shell, top with the remaining nuts and bake for 30–40 minutes until set. Cool and serve with vanilla ice cream or double cream.

PER SERVING (6) 898 kcals, protein 13g, carbs 75g, fat 63g, sat fat 19g, fibre 4g, sugar 47g, salt 0.6g

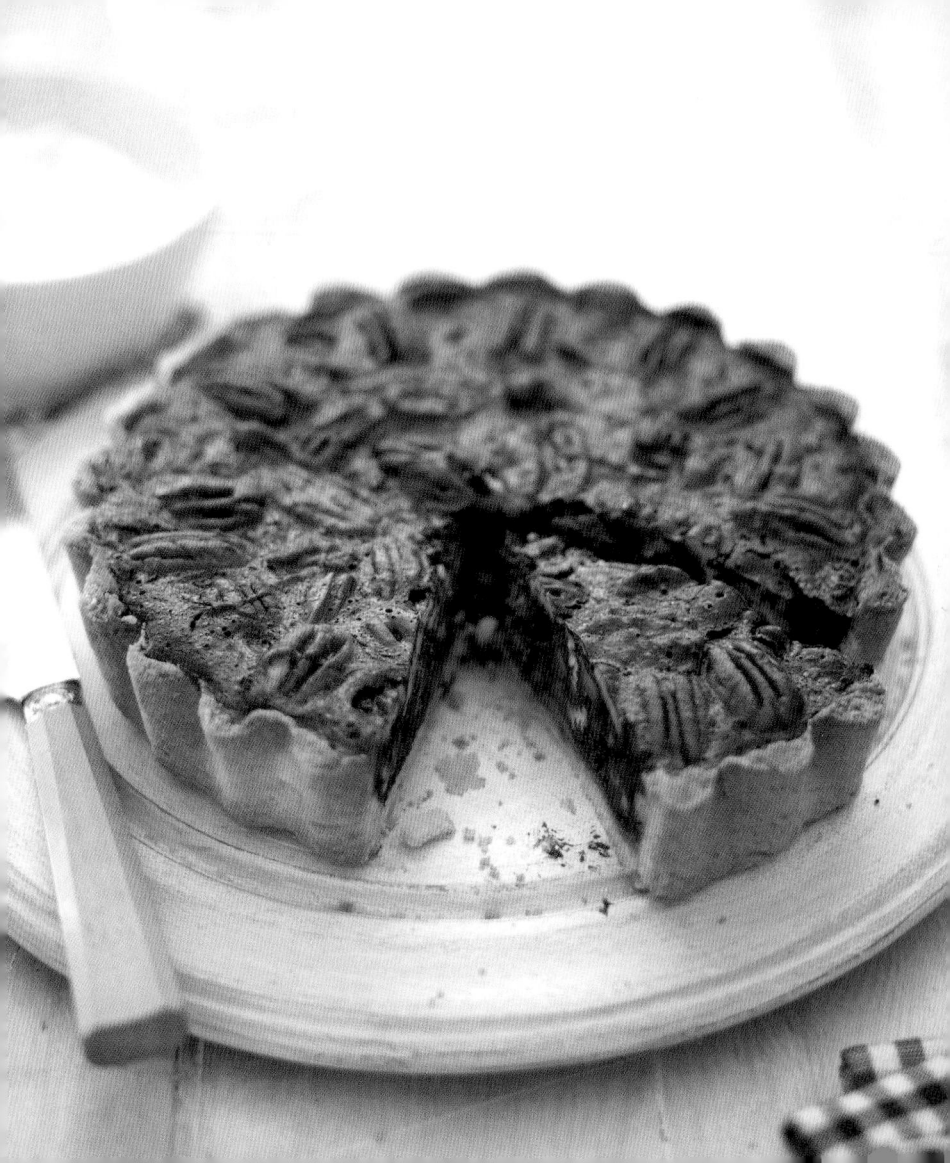

Almond & lemon meringue roulade

Crisp but squidgy almond meringue, sharp lemon-curd-marbled cream filling, and a few fresh berries to finish it off nicely.

TAKES 50 MINUTES • SERVES 6–8

4 large egg whites
225g/8oz caster sugar
1 tsp almond extract
1 tsp white wine vinegar
50g/2oz ground almonds
300ml/½ pint double cream
1–2 tbsp icing sugar
6 tbsp lemon curd
1 tbsp flaked almonds
3 strawberries, halved, to decorate

1 Heat oven to 190C/170C fan/gas 5 and line a Swiss roll tin (about 23 × 30cm) with parchment. Whisk the egg whites in a clean bowl until stiff. Slowly add the sugar, still whisking, until stiff and glossy.

2 Fold in the almond extract, vinegar and ground almonds until lightly incorporated. Pour into the tin and smooth over, tapping the tin to remove any big air bubbles.

3 Bake for 30–35 minutes or until the top is golden. Remove from the oven, cover with a sheet of baking parchment and a damp tea towel. Leave to cool.

4 When ready to serve, whip the cream until thick. Spoon a third into a piping bag and set aside. Invert the roulade on to a large sheet of parchment that has been sprinkled with icing sugar. Carefully peel off the lining paper and spread over the lemon curd, then the two-thirds of cream. Roll up carefully, using the paper to help you. Pipe the remaining cream on top of the roulade and decorate with flaked almonds and strawberry halves.

PER SERVING (8) 394 kcals, protein 4g, carbs 37g, fat 25g, sat fat 13g, fibre 0.1g, sugar 35g, salt 0.1g

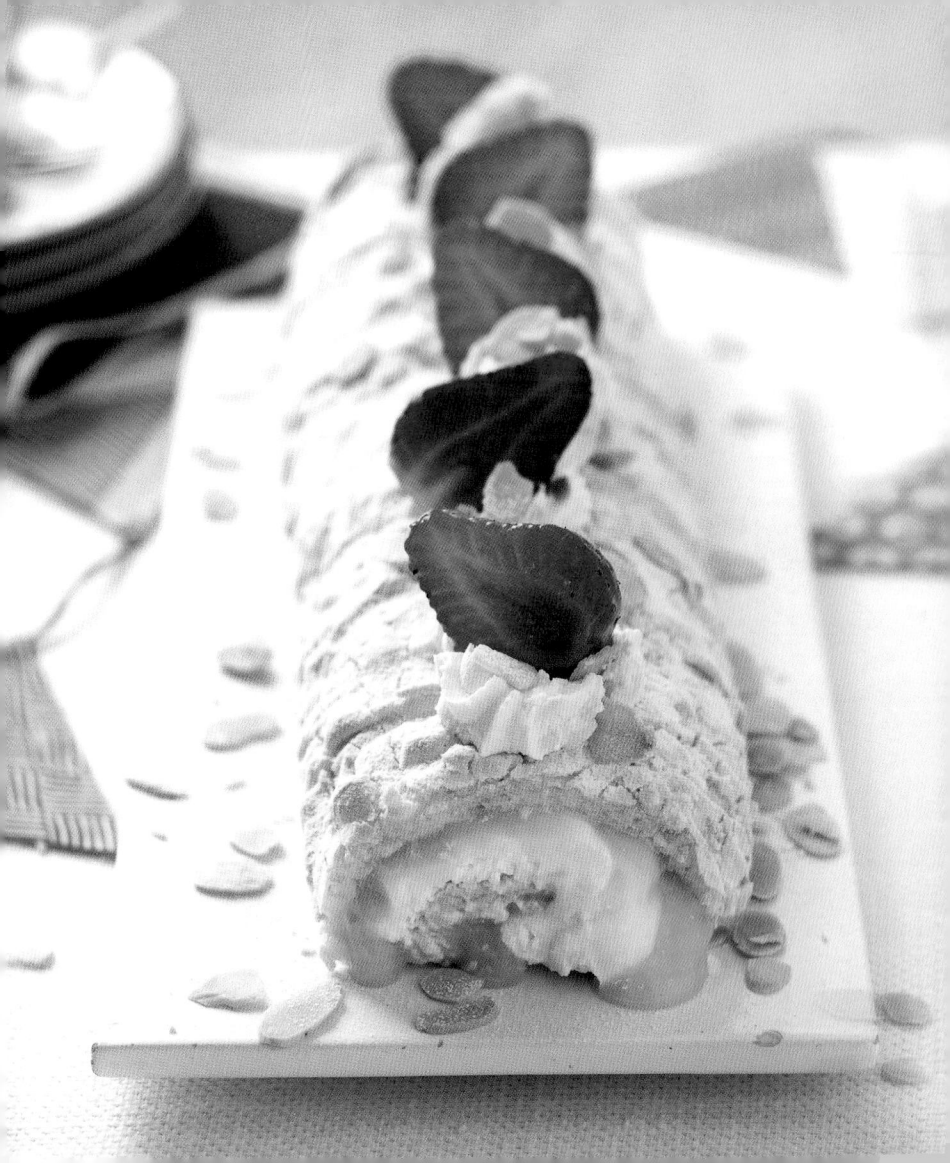

Sticky plum flapjacks

Oats don't contain gluten themselves, but during the milling process they can become contaminated; so make sure you buy a bag that states they are gluten-free.

TAKES 1½ HOURS • MAKES 18

450g/1lb plums, halved, stoned and
    roughly sliced
½ tsp ground mixed spice
300g/10oz light muscovado sugar
350g/12oz butter, plus extra for
    greasing
300g/10oz gluten-free rolled porridge
    oats
140g/5oz gluten-free plain flour
50g/2oz hazelnuts, pecan nuts or
    almonds, chopped
3 tbsp golden syrup

1 Heat oven to 200C/180C fan/gas 6. Tip the plums into a bowl. Toss with the spice, 50g/2oz of the sugar and a small pinch of salt. Set aside.

2 Gently melt the butter in a pan. In a large bowl, mix the oats, flour, nuts and remaining sugar together – making sure there are no lumps of sugar. Stir in the butter and golden syrup.

3 Grease a roughly 20cm-square baking tin. Press half the oaty mix over the base of the tin, then tip over the plums and spread to make an even layer. Press the remaining oats over the plums so they are completely covered, right to the sides of the tin. Bake for 45–50 minutes until dark golden and starting to crisp a little around the edges. Leave to cool completely, then cut into 18 pieces.

PER SERVING 335 kcals, protein 3g, carbs 38g, fat 20g, sat fat 11g, fibre 2g, sugar 22g, salt 0.34g

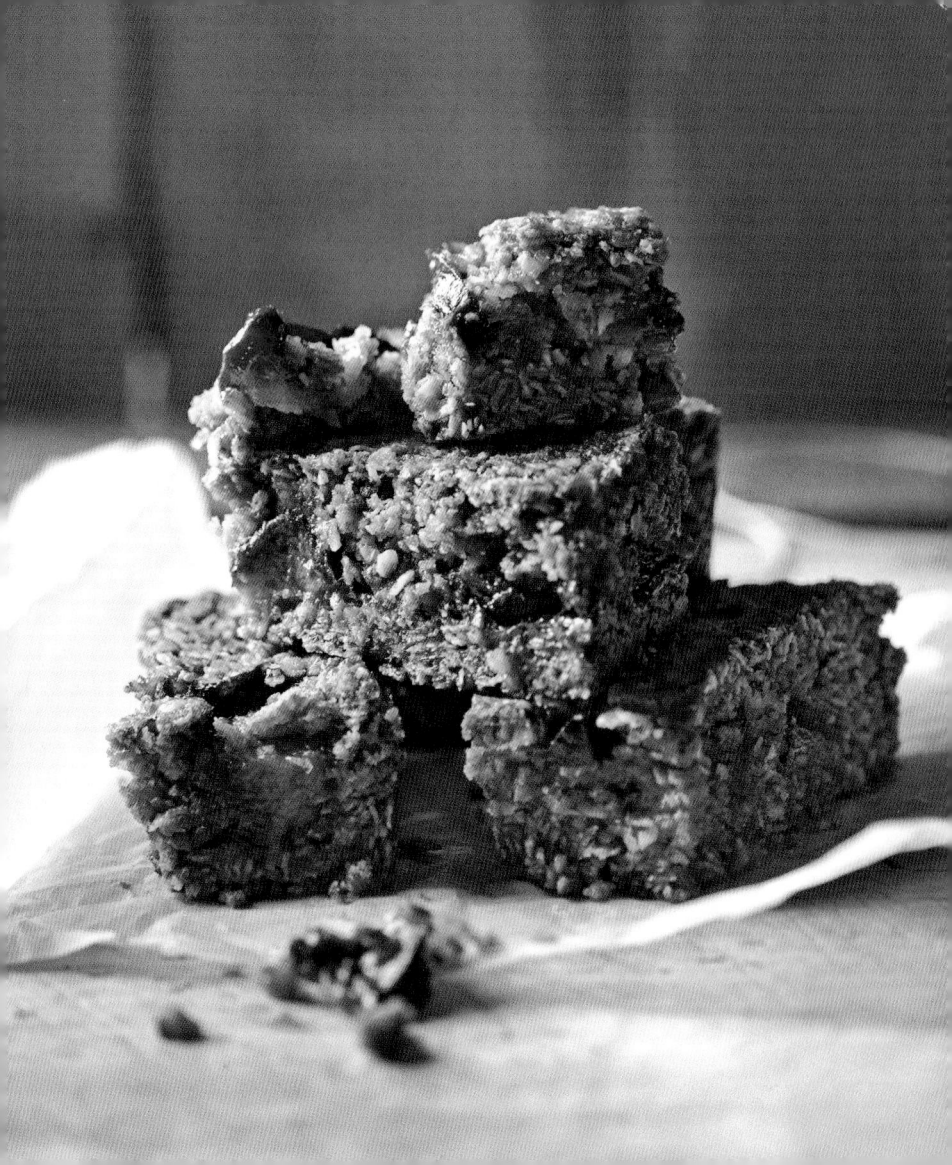

Carrot cake with cinnamon frosting

Carrot cake seems to be everybody's favourite. This loaf version is particularly easy to transport if you're going on a picnic or baking for a cake stall.

TAKES 1 HOUR 20 MINUTES, PLUS OVERNIGHT SOAKING • CUTS INTO 8–10 SLICES

zest and juice 1 orange
50g/2oz sultanas
150ml/¼ pint sunflower oil, plus extra for greasing
2 large eggs
140g/5oz light soft brown sugar
85g/3oz buckwheat flour
85g/3oz gluten-free self-raising flour (add 1 tsp xanthan gum, if it doesn't contain any)
1 tbsp ground mixed spice
1 tsp bicarbonate of soda
140g/5oz carrots, coarsely grated
50g/2oz walnuts, chopped, plus a few halves to decorate

FOR THE ICING

200g/7oz soft cheese
50g/2oz butter, softened
85g/3oz icing sugar, sifted

1 If you can, mix the orange zest and juice and sultanas the night before, or on the day simply stir the zest, juice and sultanas together and microwave on Medium for 1–2 minutes.

2 Heat oven to 180C/160C fan/gas 4 and grease and line the base and sides of a 900g loaf tin. Whisk together the oil and eggs. Mix together the sugar, flours, mixed spice and bicarb in your largest mixing bowl. Add the sultanas with any juice and zest left in the bowl, the carrots, walnuts and whisked egg mixture to the dry ingredients, then thoroughly mix. Tip into the loaf tin and bake for 1 hour, or until an inserted skewer comes out clean. Cool the cake in the tin.

3 With an electric whisk, beat together the soft cheese, butter and icing sugar until smooth. Spread over the top of the cake and decorate with walnut halves.

PER SERVING (8) 592 kcals, protein 7g, carbs 51g, fat 41g, sat fat 14g, fibre 2g, sugar 36g, salt 0.83g

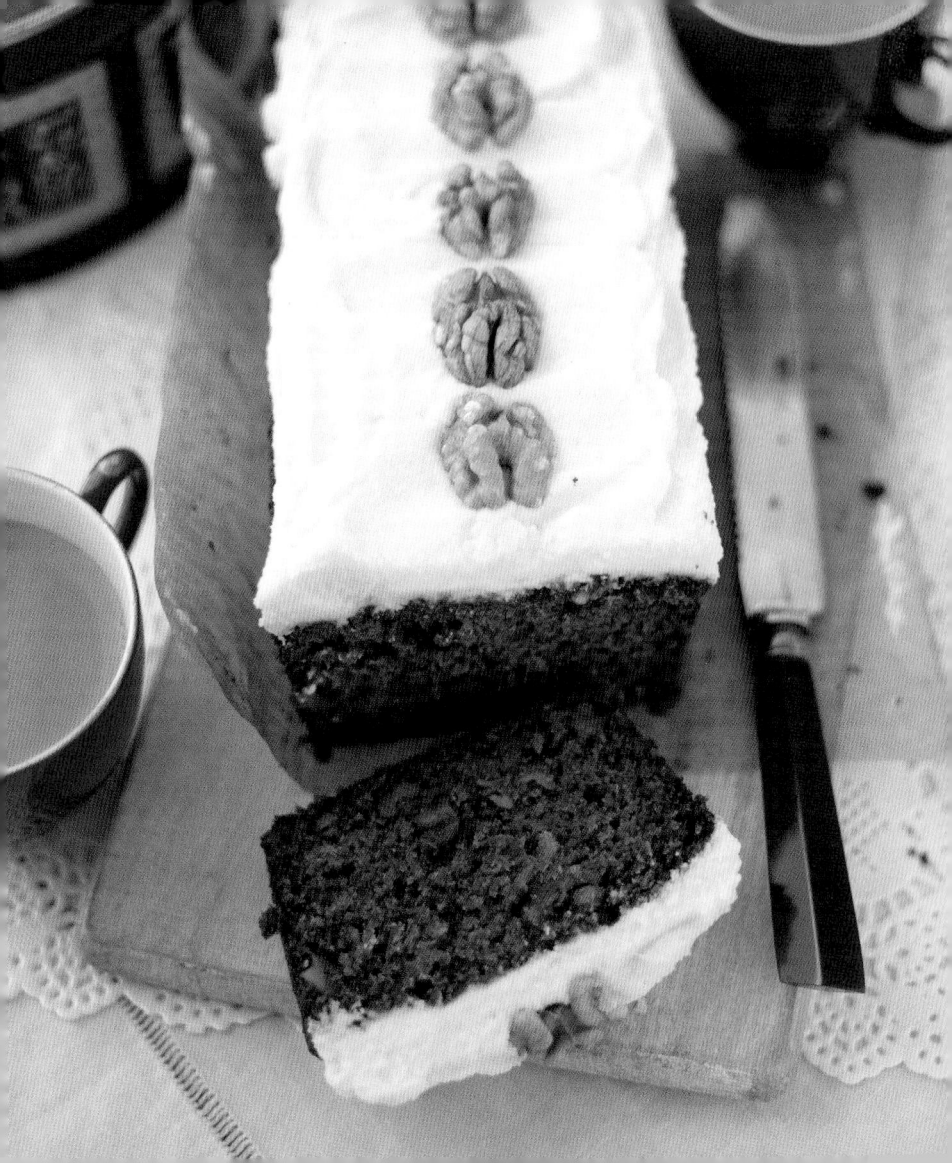

Chocolate & Earl Grey torte

Entertaining has never been so easy: this gorgeous fudgy torte is completely make-ahead, but sophisticated enough to really impress.

TAKES 1 HOUR, PLUS COOLING

● **SERVES 8**

leaves from 2 Earl Grey tea bags
100ml/3½fl oz hot milk
250g/9oz good-quality dark chocolate
  (we used 78% cocoa solids)
200g/7oz butter, diced
140g/5oz ground almonds
6 eggs, separated
200g/7oz caster sugar
cocoa powder and icing sugar, to dust
crème fraîche or cream, to serve

1 Heat oven to 180C/160C fan/gas 4. Grease and line the base and sides of a deep 22cm-round loose-bottomed tin with baking parchment, so the paper comes about 2.5cm/1in above the sides. Stir the Earl Grey tea into the hot milk.

2 Melt the chocolate, butter and a pinch of salt together in a bowl over a pan of barely simmering water. Then stir in the ground almonds, followed by the egg yolks and milky tea, including the leaves. Beat the egg whites until stiff, then beat in the caster sugar until stiff-ish again. Fold the whites through the chocolate mix and scrape into the tin. Bake for 30–35 minutes – it should still have a slight wobble. Then cool completely in the tin.

3 Carefully remove from the tin and lift on to a serving plate. Dust all over with cocoa and icing sugar, then serve in slices with crème fraîche or cream.

PER SERVING 514 kcals, protein 10g, carbs 34g, fat 37g, sat fat 17g, fibre 3g, sugar 29g, salt 0.39g

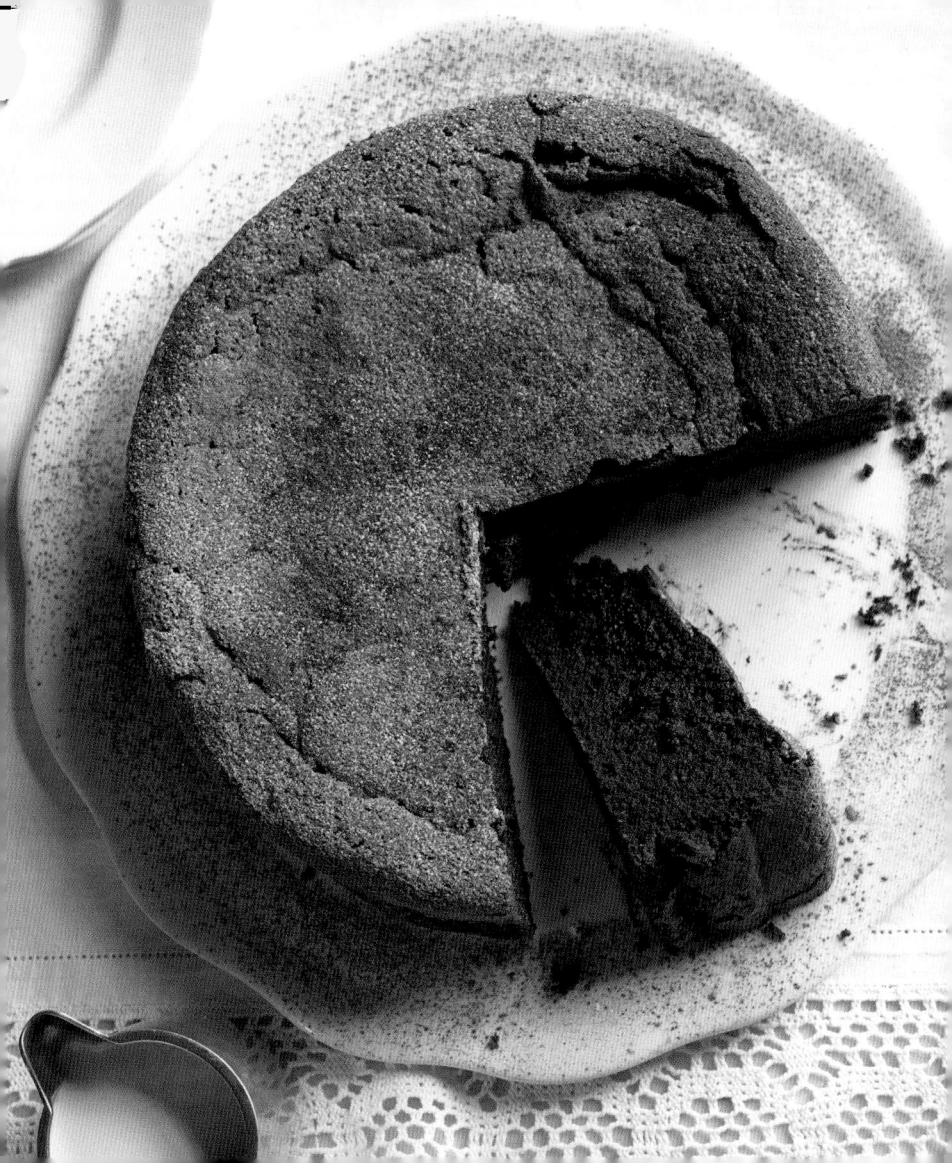

Lemon & poppy seed cupcakes

You'll love these little cakes – delicate and lemony, made modern with the addition of toasted poppy seeds.

TAKES 1 HOUR, PLUS COOLING
● **MAKES 12**

120g/4½oz gluten-free self-raising flour (add 1 tsp xanthan gum, if it doesn't contain any)

100g/4oz ground almonds

175g/6oz golden caster sugar

zest 2 lemons

1 tbsp poppy seeds, toasted

3 large eggs

100g/4oz natural yogurt

175g/6oz butter, melted and cooled a little

FOR THE ICING AND DECORATION

225g/8oz butter, softened

400g/14oz icing sugar, sifted

juice 1 lemon

few drops yellow food colouring, icing flowers or yellow sprinkles, to decorate

1 Heat oven to 180C/160C fan/gas 4. Line a 12-hole muffin tin with paper cases. Mix the flour, almonds, sugar, lemon zest and poppy seeds in a bowl. Beat the eggs into the yogurt, then tip into the dry ingredients with the butter. Mix together until lump-free, then divide among the cases. Bake for 20 minutes until a skewer poked in comes out clean. Leave to cool.

2 To ice, beat the butter until soft, then gradually beat in the icing sugar and lemon juice. Stir in enough food colouring for a pale lemon colour, then spoon into a piping bag with a large star nozzle.

3 Ice each cake, holding the piping bag almost upright with the nozzle about 1cm/½in from the surface of the cake. Pipe one spiral of icing around the edge, then pause to break the flow then move the nozzle towards the centre and pipe a second smaller spiral that continues until there are no gaps. Slightly 'dot' the nozzle into the icing as you stop squeezing to finish neatly. Top with decorations.

PER CUPCAKE 529 kcals, protein 4g, carbs 66g, fat 30g, sat fat 18g, fibre 1g, sugar 51g, salt 0.75g

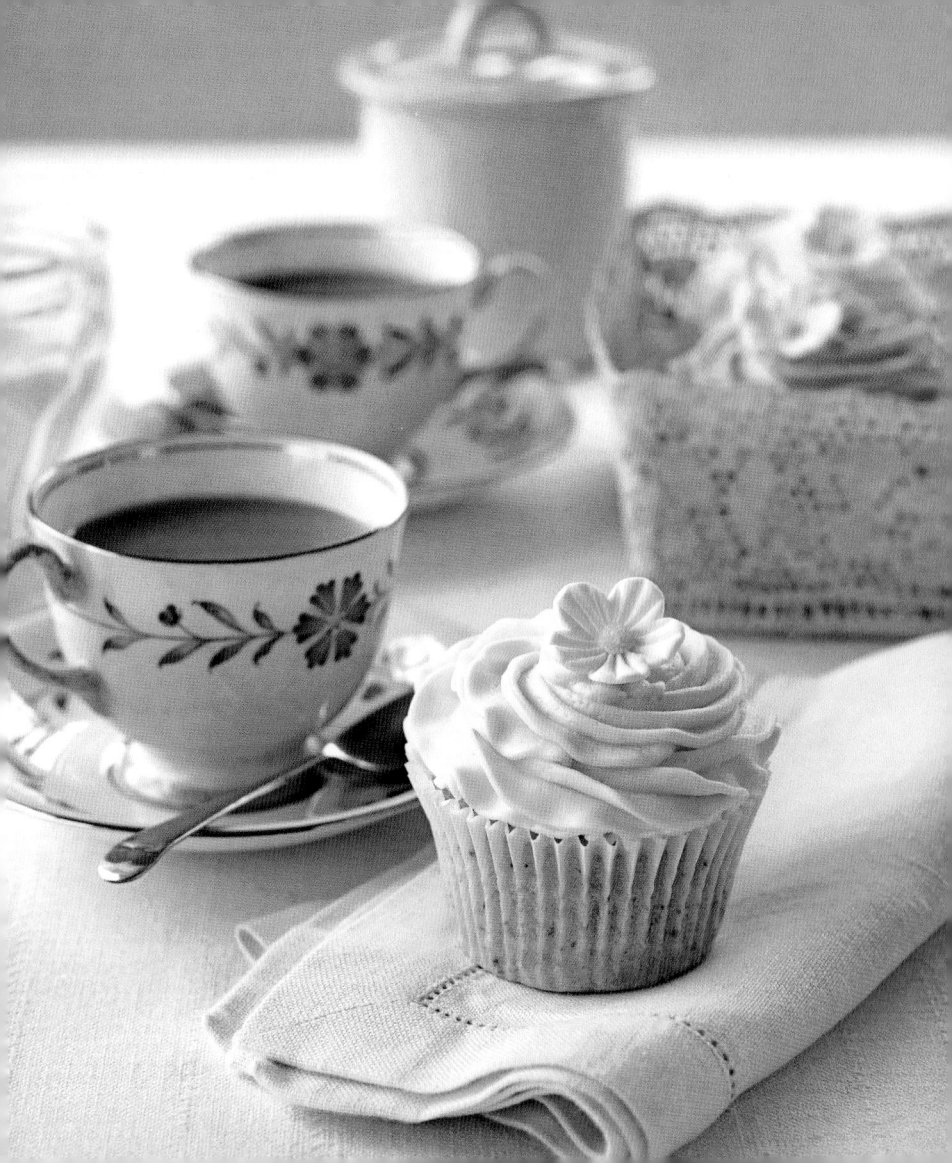

Cranberry & cream cheese muffins

These are particularly delicious on Christmas morning – pass them round while the kids are opening their presents.

TAKES 40 MINUTES, PLUS COOLING
- **MAKES 12**

100g/4oz soft cheese

250g/9oz caster sugar

175g/6oz cranberries

200g/7oz gluten-free plain flour

2 tsp gluten-free baking powder

2 tsp xanthan gum

2 large eggs

75ml/2½fl oz flavourless oil, such as sunflower

1 tsp vanilla extract

1 Heat oven to 190C/170C fan/gas 5. Line a 12-hole muffin tin with muffin cases. Beat the soft cheese with 25g/1oz of the sugar and chill until needed. Heat the cranberries together with another 25g/1oz of the sugar until they start to pop. Mash lightly and cool.

2 Sift the flour into a large bowl and add the remaining sugar, baking powder, xanthan gum and a pinch of salt. Add the eggs, oil, vanilla and cranberry mixture, and stir together. Don't worry if the mix looks a bit lumpy. Divide it among the cases; they should look about two-thirds full. Make a small dip in the centre of each and put a blob of soft cheese in. Bake for 25 minutes or until risen and golden. Cool on a wire rack.

PER MUFFIN 230 kcals, protein 3g, carbs 36g, fat 9g, sat fat 2g, fibre 1g, sugar 23g, salt 0.33g

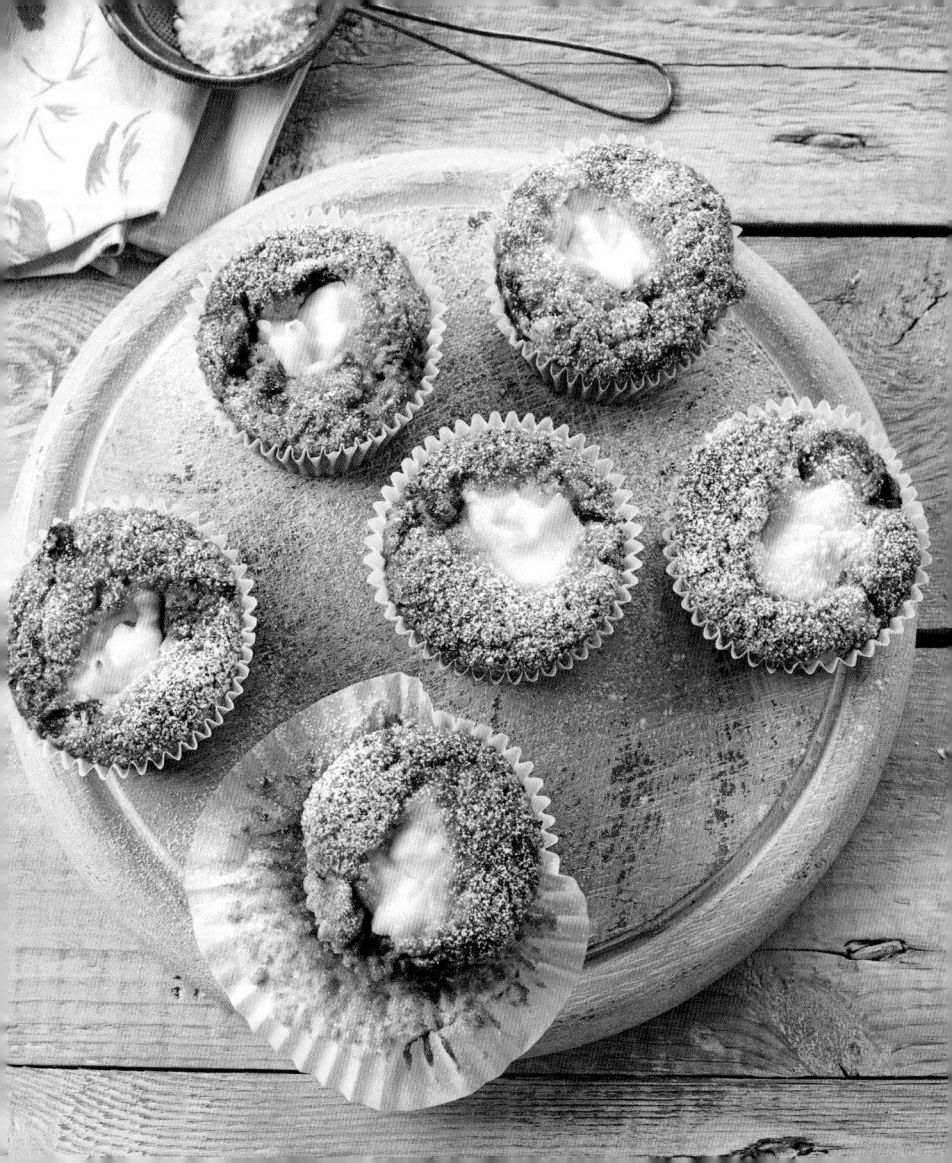

Toasted cumin flatbreads

Whether you're cooking an Indian curry or a Moroccan tagine, these super-simple breads will be ideal alongside, and are perfect for mopping up tasty sauces or dips.

TAKES 20 MINUTES ● MAKES 8

400g/14oz gluten-free self-raising flour, plus extra for dusting
1 tbsp cumin seeds, toasted
300g/10oz natural yogurt

1 Heat the grill to a low setting and dust a baking sheet with a little flour. Mix the flour and cumin seeds in a bowl, then season. Stir in the yogurt and 100ml/3½fl oz water, then mix well to form a soft dough.

2 Divide the dough into eight equal pieces, then shape into circles or ovals about 0.5cm/¼in thick. Dust lightly with a little flour. Grill on the baking sheet for 3–5 minutes on each side until golden and puffed. Serve warm.

PER FLATBREAD 200 kcals, protein 5g, carbs 47g, fat 2g, sat fat none, fibre 1g, sugar 2g, salt 0.08g

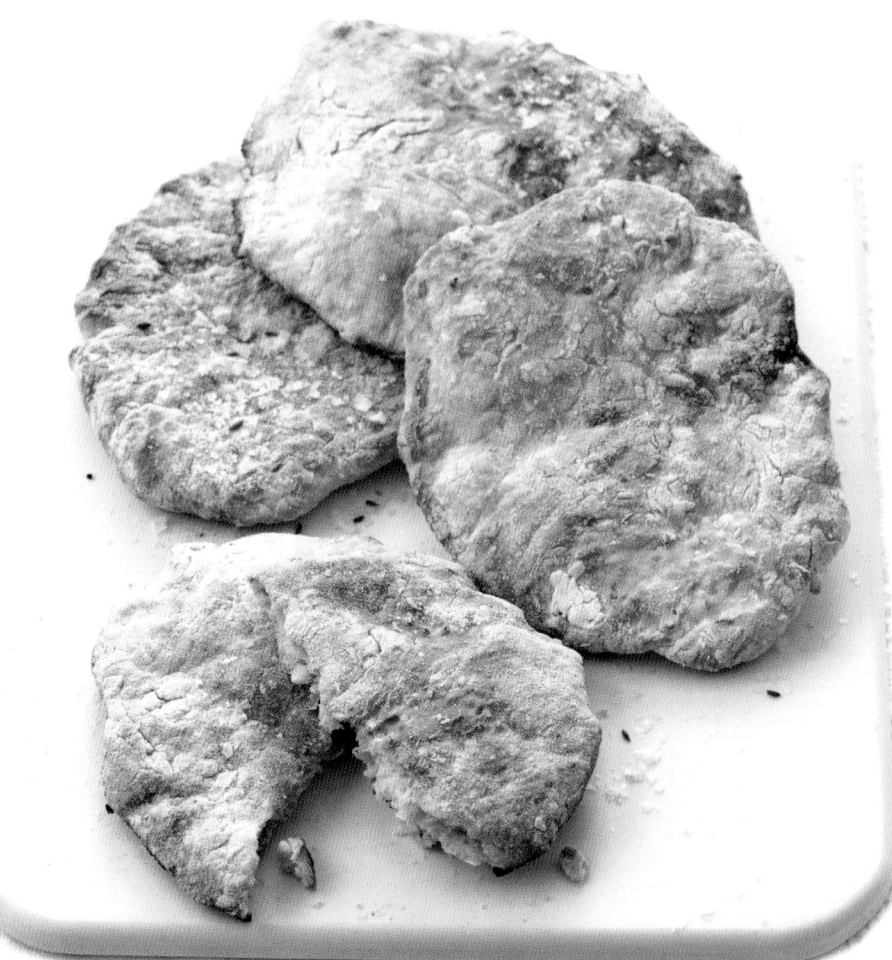

Cheese scones

A fresh-from-the-oven warm cheese scone, spread with butter and onion chutney, might just be the best thing in the whole wide world.

TAKES 40 MINUTES • **MAKES 8–10**

200g/7oz gluten-free self-raising flour (add 2 tsp xanthan gum, if it doesn't contain any), plus extra for rolling
1 tsp bicarbonate of soda
50g/2oz cold butter, cubed, plus extra to serve
100g/4oz Cheddar, grated
150ml/¼ pint buttermilk
1 egg, beaten
onion chutney, to serve

1 Heat oven to 220C/200C fan/gas 7. Line a baking sheet with baking parchment. Sift the flour, bicarb and a pinch of salt in a food processor, then add the butter and blitz until it resembles breadcrumbs.

2 Tip the mixture into a large bowl, then stir in 85g/3oz of the cheese. Add the buttermilk, mixing together with a cutlery knife to form a dough.

3 Turn out on to a floured surface and lightly bring together quickly, then flatten the dough with your hands to about 3cm/1¼in thickness. Using a roughly 6cm cutter, cut out rounds of the dough, gently rolling any scraps together and re-cutting.

4 Put the scones on the prepared baking sheet and brush the tops with a little egg. Scatter over the remaining cheese and bake for 12–14 minutes until golden. Eat warm.

PER SCONE (8) 178 kcals, protein 5g, carbs 19g, fat 9g, sat fat 5g, fibre 1g, sugar 3g, salt 0.7g

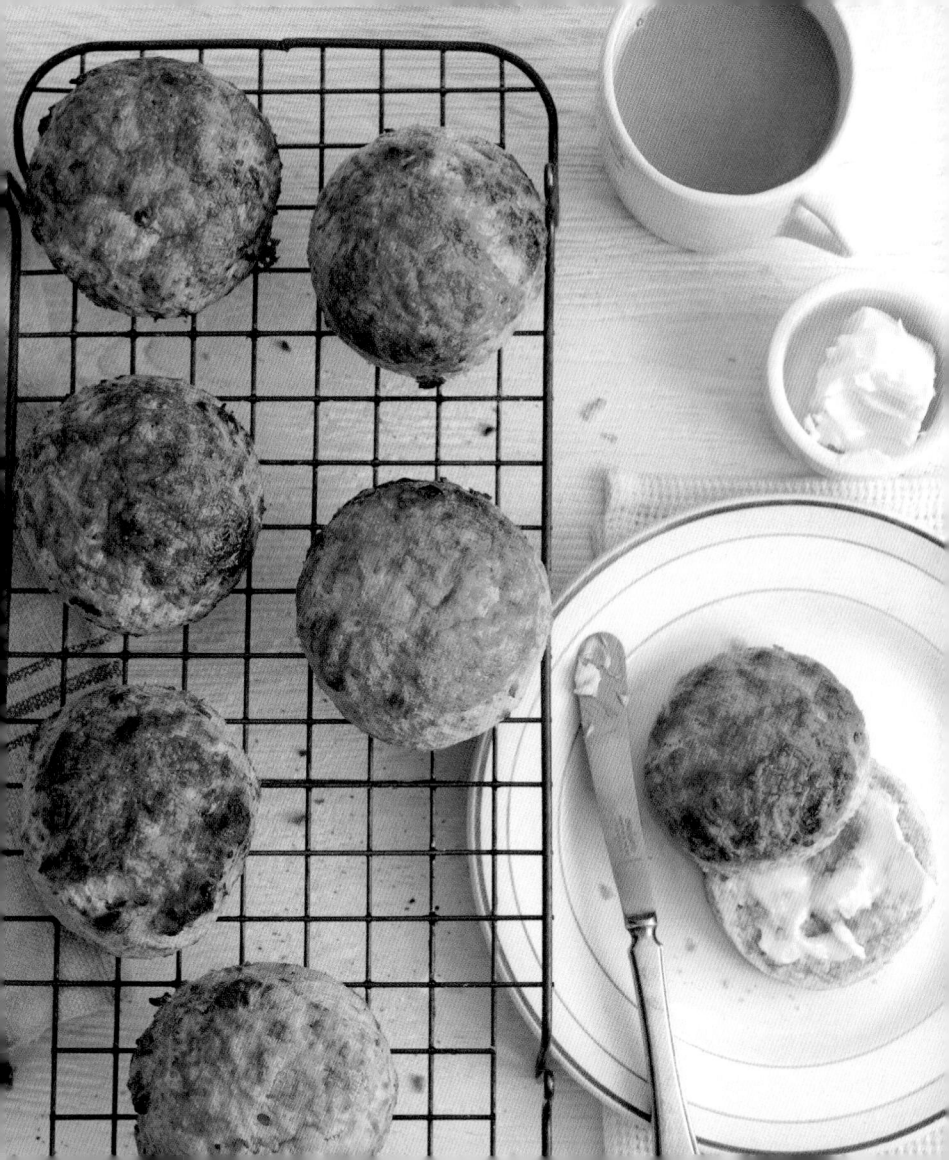

Cornbread muffins

Serve with a beef chilli or spicy tomato soup, or simply on their own, warm, spread with lots of butter or cream cheese.

TAKES 1 HOUR • MAKES 12

85g/3oz melted butter, plus extra knob
    for frying
1 large sweetcorn, kernels sliced off
1 small onion, finely chopped
½ red chilli, deseeded and finely
    chopped
140g/5oz gluten-free plain flour
140g/5oz polenta or cornmeal
2 tsp gluten-free baking powder
1 tsp xanthan gum
50g/2oz strong Cheddar or vegetarian
    alternative, grated
2 eggs
284ml pot buttermilk
100ml/3½fl oz milk

1 Heat oven to 200C/180C fan/gas 6 and brush a 12-hole muffin tin with some of the melted butter. Put the corn kernels in a pan with the onion, chilli and the extra knob of butter. Gently fry for 5–10 minutes until golden and soft.
2 Mix together the flour, polenta or cornmeal, baking powder, xanthan gum and Cheddar or vegetarian alternative with 1 teaspoon salt in a large mixing bowl. Whisk together the eggs, buttermilk and milk, then stir into the dry ingredients with the remaining melted butter and the corn mixture. Divide among the muffin holes (they will be quite full) and bake for 25–30 minutes or until golden brown and cooked through – poke in a skewer to check. Best eaten warm on the day.

PER MUFFIN 189 kcals, protein 6g, carbs 22g, fat 9g, sat fat 5g, fibre 1g, sugar 3g, salt 0.44g

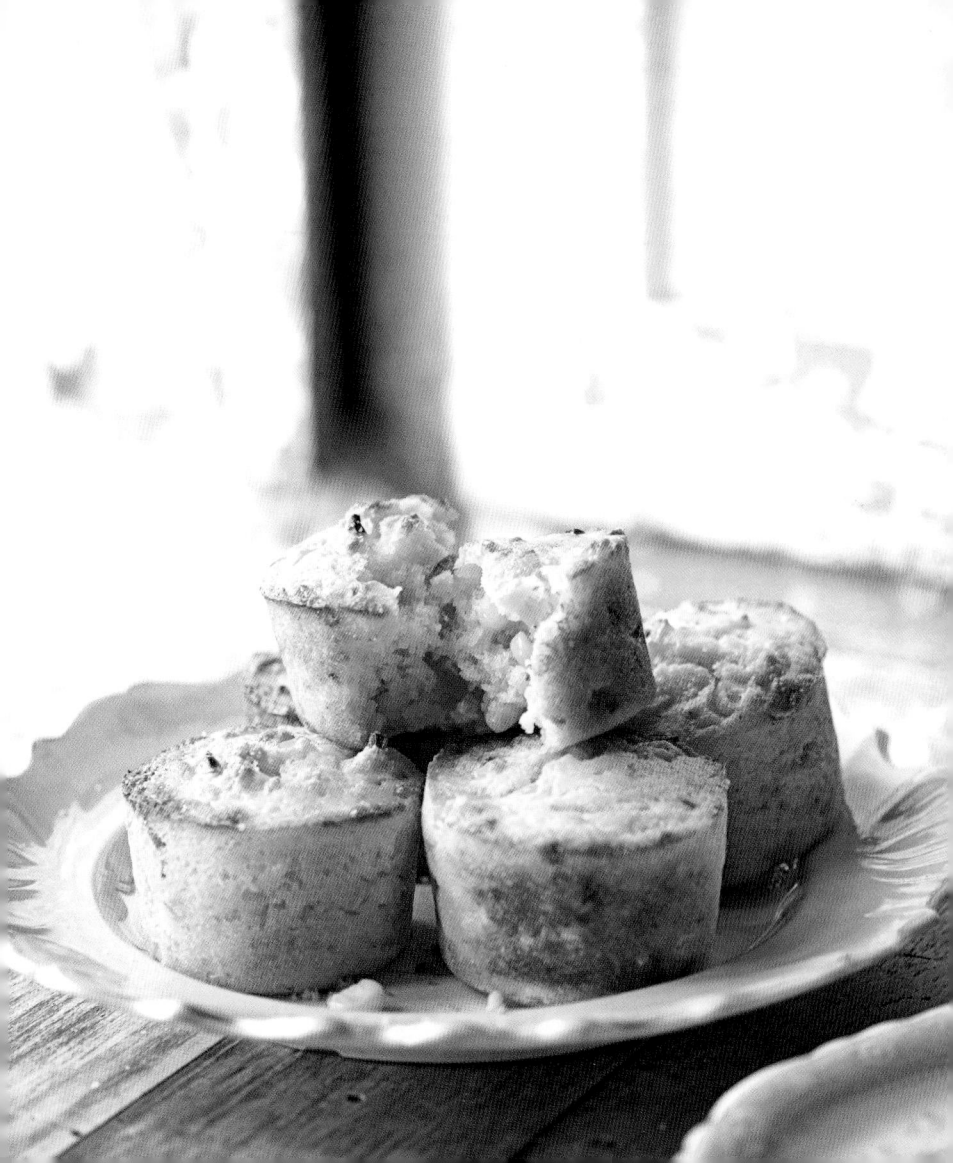

Dill scones

For taller scones, dip the cutter into flour each time you use it. The flour will stop the cutter from sticking and squashing down the edges of the dough.

TAKES 45 MINUTES ● MAKES 7–8

200g/7oz gluten-free plain flour, plus extra for dusting

200g/7oz buckwheat flour

1 tsp bicarbonate of soda

½ × 20g pack dill, finely chopped

50g/2oz unsalted butter, very cold and cut into cubes

300ml/½ pint milk, warmed, plus extra for brushing

1 tsp poppy seeds

1 Heat oven to 230C/210C fan/gas 8 and lightly flour a baking sheet. Mix the flours, bicarb, chopped dill and 1 teaspoon salt in a large bowl, then rub in the butter until it disappears. Tip in the milk and stir briefly to a sticky dough.

2 Scrape the dough on to a floured surface, dust it and your hands with more flour, then fold the dough over 2–3 times to smooth a little. Pat into a 4cm/1½in-deep round. Use a 7cm cutter to stamp out scones. Press the trimmings together and repeat. Brush with milk, scatter with poppy seeds, then bake for 15–18 minutes or until golden and well risen. Cool on a wire rack. As with all scones, these are best eaten on the day they are made.

PER SCONE 365 kcals, protein 21g, carbs 48g, fat 10g, sat fat 5g, fibre 4g, sugar 7g, salt 2.85g

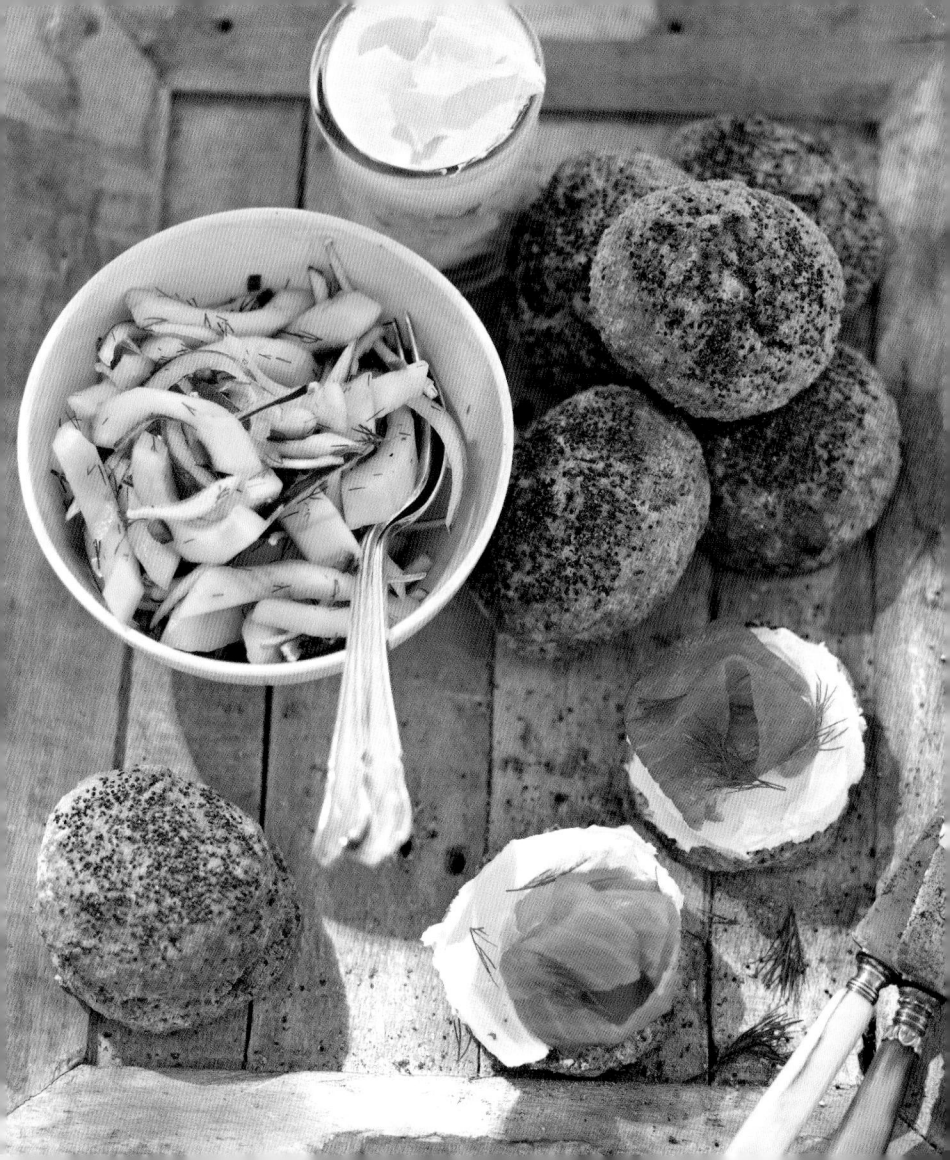

Polenta & pancetta stuffing

This creamy stuffing is really unusual, but absolutely delicious – serve it with roast chicken and you won't miss the classic breadcrumb stuffing one bit.

TAKES 1 HOUR 20 MINUTES

● **SERVES 8**

1 onion, finely chopped
2 tbsp olive oil
2 × 70g packs cubetti di pancetta
1 garlic clove, crushed
2 thyme sprigs, leaves stripped and
  finely chopped, plus extra to garnish
500g pack ready-cooked polenta,
  chopped into cubes
50g/2oz Parmesan, grated
250ml/9fl oz single or whipping cream
250ml/9fl oz chicken or vegetable stock
  made with gluten-free stock cubes

1 Heat oven to 200C/180C fan/gas 6. In a large frying pan, gently fry the onion in the oil until soft, about 8–10 minutes. Stir in the pancetta, garlic and thyme, and cook until the pancetta is browned and crisp. Stir in the polenta and half the cheese, and cook for a few minutes – don't worry if the polenta breaks up. You can prepare to this stage up to a day ahead.

2 Add the cream and stock to the pan, mix thoroughly, then pour into an oiled baking dish. Sprinkle over the remaining cheese and bake for 40 minutes or until browned on top. Allow to stand for 10 minutes before serving with an extra garnish of thyme.

PER SERVING 268 kcals, protein 12g, carbs 12g, fat 19g, sat fat 9g, fibre 2g, sugar 3g, salt 2.19g

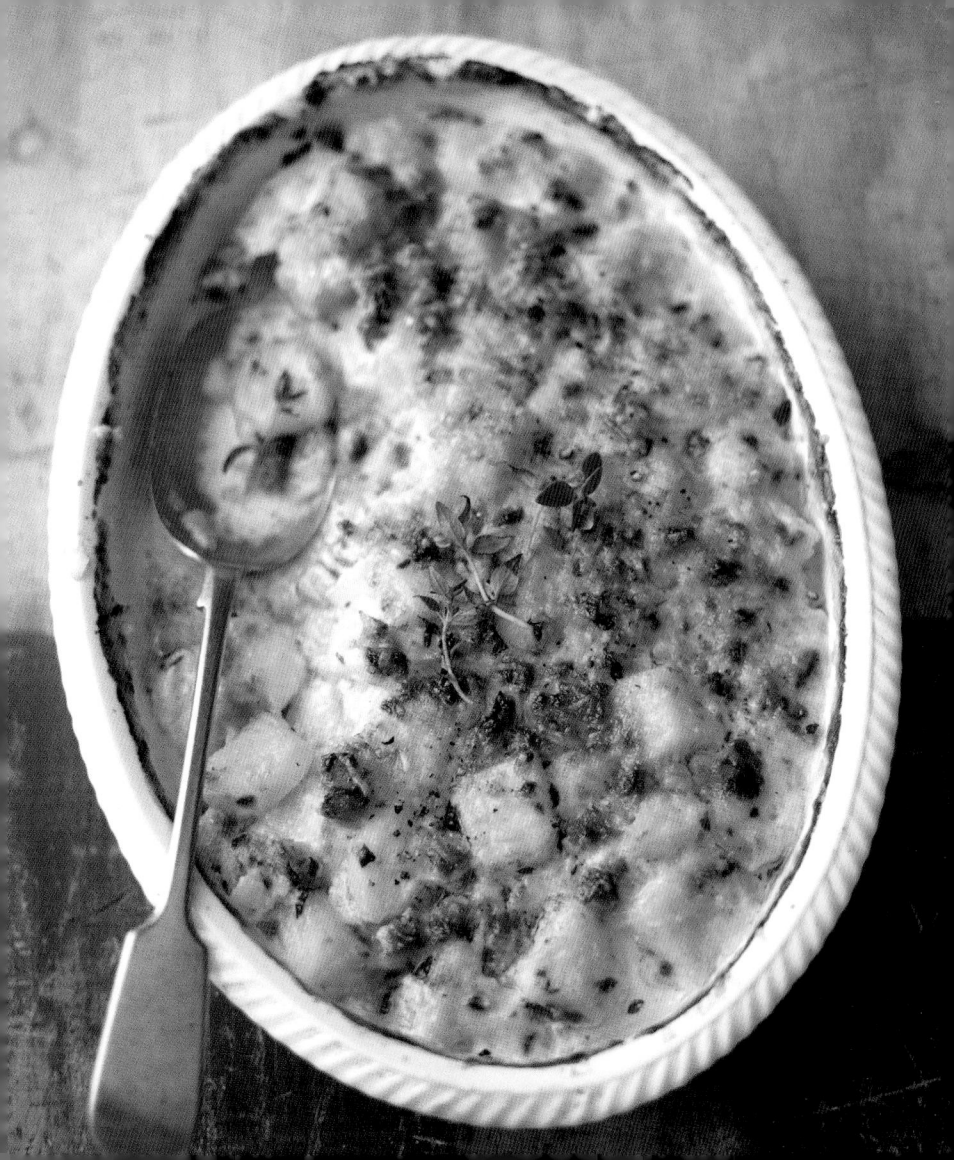

Blue cheese & walnut rolls

Blue cheese pairs very well with the walnuts in these rolls, but any cheese would work quite nicely – or even a mixture, if you're using up scraps from the fridge.

TAKES 50 MINUTES • MAKES 8

200g/7oz cornflour

200g/7oz buckwheat flour, plus extra for rolling

85g/3oz potato starch

2 tbsp soya flour

2 tsp xanthan gum

7g sachet easy-bake dried yeast

1 tbsp caster sugar

5 tbsp natural yogurt

2 tbsp olive oil, plus extra for greasing

1 tbsp white wine vinegar

140g/5oz walnuts, finely chopped in a food processor

250g/9oz blue cheese such as Roquefort, crumbled

2 medium eggs, beaten

1 Mix the flours, potato starch, soya flour, xanthan gum, yeast, sugar and 1½ teaspoon salt in a bowl. Measure 400ml/14fl oz hand-warm water, then stir in the yogurt, olive oil and vinegar. Mix into the dry ingredients until a soft dough comes together. Cover loosely with some oiled cling film and leave to rise for an hour somewhere warm-ish.

2 Knead in the walnuts. Tip the dough out on to a lightly floured surface and roll out into a rectangle, about 50 × 20cm/20 × 8in, 1cm/½in thick. Sprinkle the blue cheese over the dough and lightly press in. Put the rectangle widthways in front of you and roll up like a Swiss roll. Cut into eight equal-sized pieces and put them on to a lightly greased baking sheet, cut-side down. Cover with cling film and leave to rise for 1 hour.

3 Heat oven to 240C/220C fan/gas 9. Brush each roll with the beaten egg and bake for 20 minutes. Leave to cool for a few minutes and eat while still warm.

PER ROLL 492 kcals, protein 18g, carbs 46g, fat 27g, sat fat 10g, fibre 3g, sugar 1g, salt 1.42g

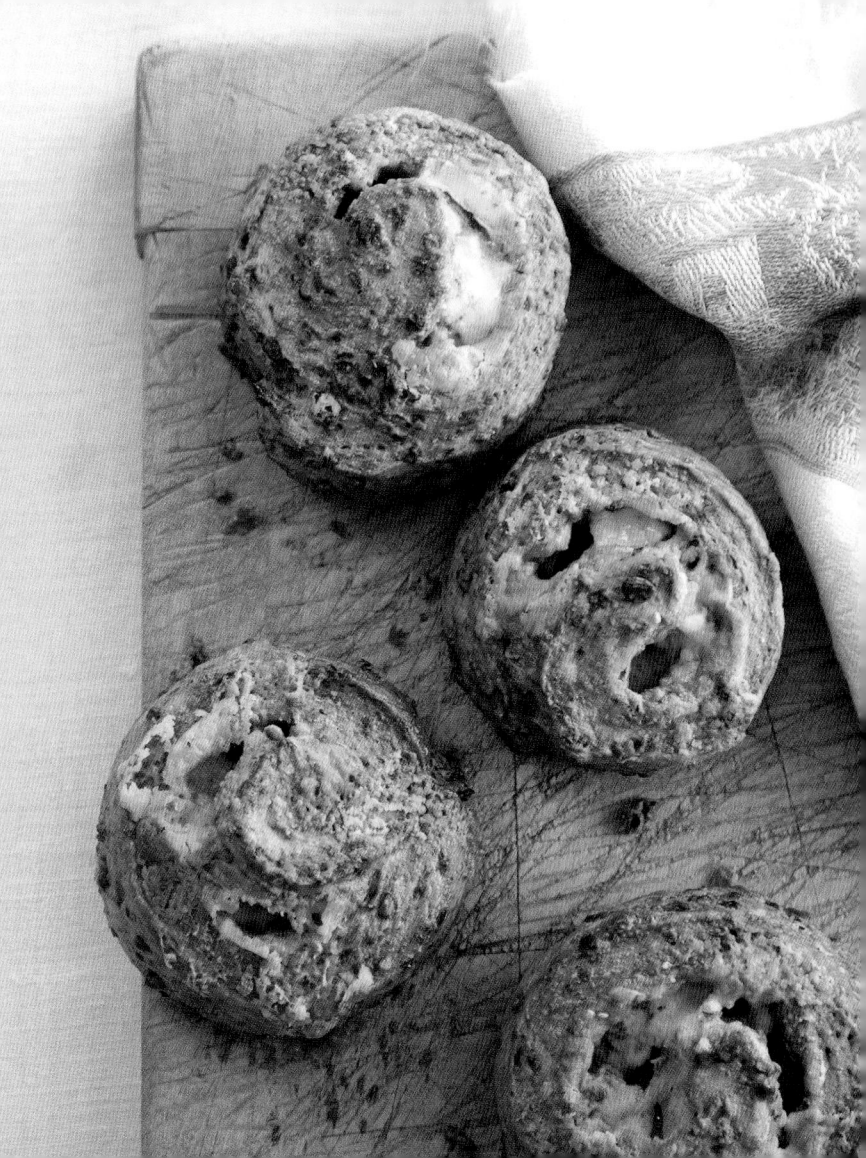

Malted walnut–seed loaf

This dense, seeded loaf is absolutely delicious. Try it alongside a big bowl of soup, then spread jam and butter over toasted leftovers for breakfast the next morning.

TAKES 1¼ HOURS, PLUS RISING
- **CUTS INTO 12 SLICES**

100g/4oz cornflour

300g/10oz gluten-free brown bread flour

85g/3oz potato starch

2 tbsp soya flour

2 tsp xanthan gum

7g sachet easy-bake dried yeast

1 tbsp caster sugar

450ml/16fl oz milk, warmed to hand temperature

2 tbsp sunflower oil, plus extra for greasing

1 tbsp white wine vinegar

100g/4oz mixed seeds (we used linseeds, hemp seeds, pumpkin seeds and sesame seeds)

50g/2oz walnuts, roughly chopped

1 Mix the flours, potato starch, soya flour, xanthan gum, yeast, sugar and 1½ teaspoon salt in a large bowl. Mix the milk, oil and vinegar and stir into the dry ingredients until a soft dough comes together. Cover loosely with some oiled cling film and leave to rise for an hour somewhere warm-ish.

2 Knead in most of the seeds and the walnuts. Shape into a large round – oiled hands will help. Roll the round in the remaining seeds, then lift the bread on to a lightly oiled baking sheet. Loosely cover again with oiled cling film and leave for another hour.

3 Heat oven to 220C/200C fan/gas 7. Bake the bread for 15 minutes, then reduce the heat to 190C/170C fan/gas 5 and continue to bake for 30 minutes until the loaf sounds hollow when tapped on the base. Leave the bread on a wire rack to cool, wrapped in a clean tea towel.

PER SLICE 172 kcals, protein 7g, carbs 28g, fat 4g, sat fat 1g, fibre 5g, sugar 1g, salt 0.43g

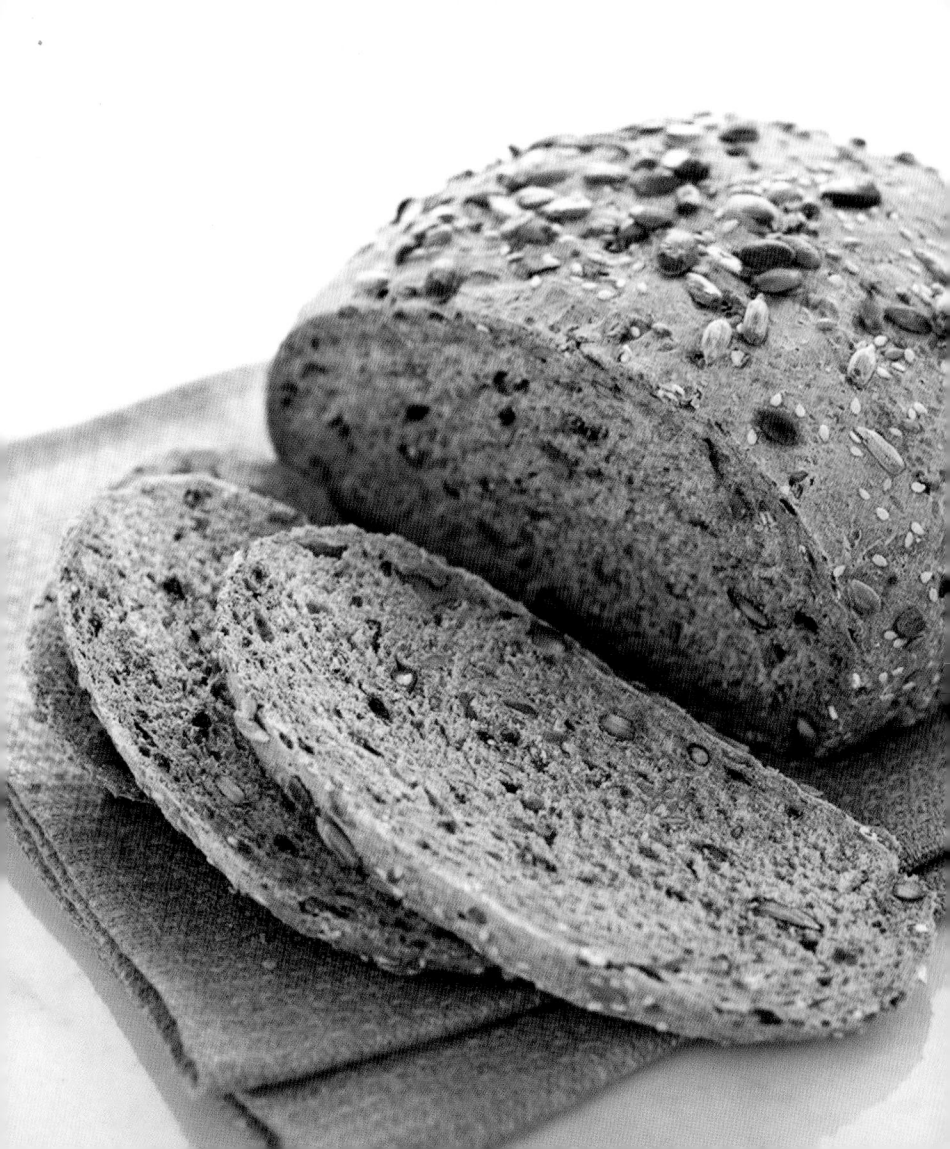

Spiced veggie Scotch eggs

You'll love the modern flavour-twist on these vegetarian versions of a British classic. If you like your treats a little spicier, swap the korma paste for something with more kick.

TAKES 45 MINUTES • MAKES 6

7 large eggs
2 tbsp olive oil
1 onion, chopped
250g/9oz grated carrot
2 heaped tbsp gluten-free korma curry paste
200g/7oz gluten-free wholemeal bread, whizzed into crumbs
85g/3oz roasted cashew nuts, finely chopped

1 Put 6 of the eggs in a pan of cold water and bring to the boil. Boil for 5 minutes, then cool quickly in cold water. Carefully peel off the shells.

2 While the eggs are cooling, heat the oil, fry the onion for 5 minutes, then add the carrot and cook for 10 minutes more until soft. Stir in the curry paste and fry for a few minutes more. Stir in the bread, then, when the mixture is cool, beat the remaining egg and stir in with some seasoning to make a paste.

3 Divide the paste into six and flatten with your hands (wetting them makes this a bit easier), then use to wrap round each egg – the mixture will seal well as you press it together. Roll in the cashews and chill until ready to cook. The prepared eggs can be kept in the fridge overnight.

4 Heat oven to 190C/170C fan/gas 5, then bake the eggs for 15–20 minutes. Cool for 5 minutes, then carefully cut in half using a very sharp knife.

PER EGG 340 kcals, protein 15g, carbs 24g, fat 21g, sat fat 4g, fibre 3g, sugar 6g, salt 0.77g

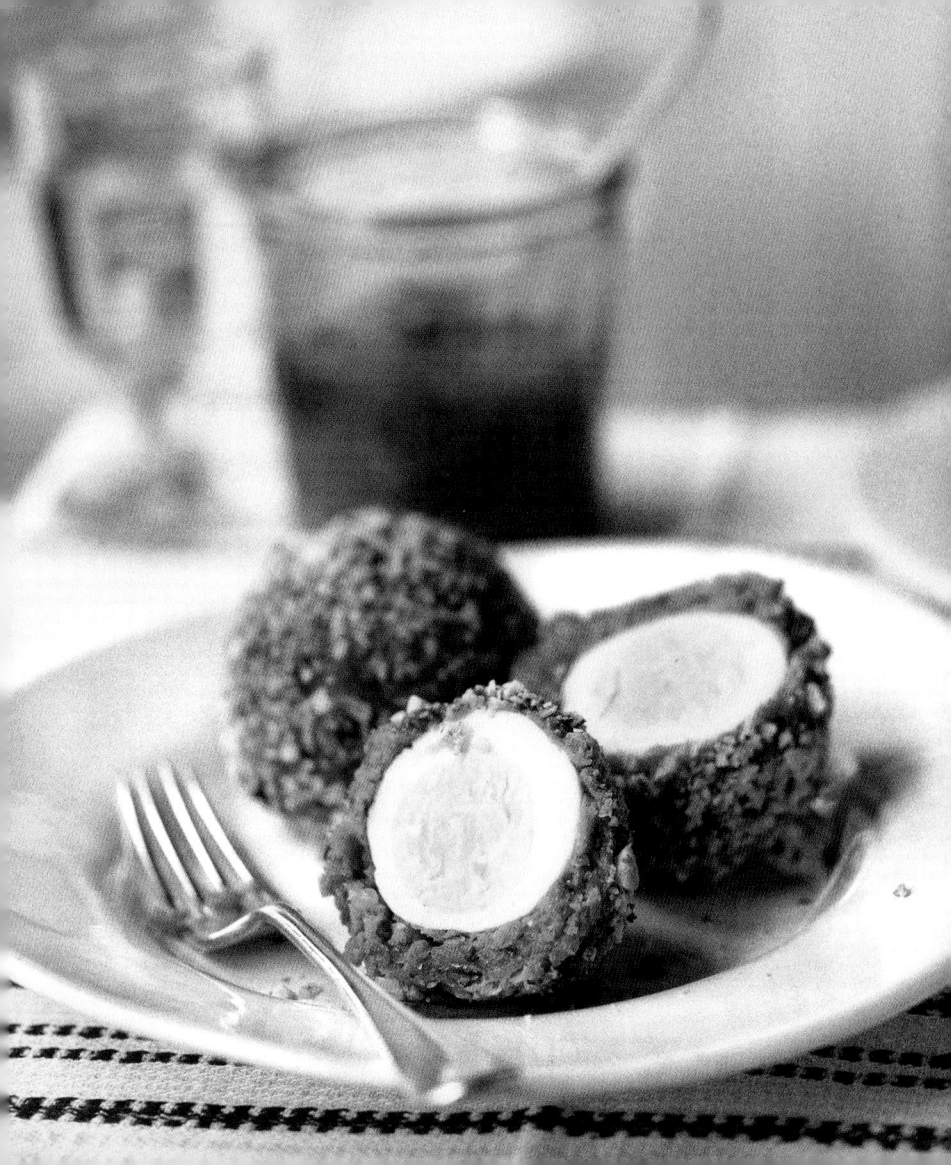

Foccaccia rolls

These flavoured breads are delicious instead of a sandwich, or serve them alongside pasta and vary the toppings to complement your dish.

TAKES 1 HOUR, PLUS RISING
- **MAKES 6**

400g/14oz cornflour
85g/3oz potato starch
2 tbsp soya flour
2 tsp xanthan gum
7g sachet easy-bake dried yeast
1 tbsp caster sugar
5 tbsp natural yogurt
2 tbsp olive oil, plus extra for greasing and drizzling
1 tbsp white wine vinegar
100g/4oz roasted peppers from a jar, sliced
85g/3oz Camembert or similar, diced
20 small black olives
handful rocket leaves
good pinch dried oregano

1 Mix the cornflour, potato starch, soya flour, xanthan gum, yeast, sugar and 1½ teaspoons salt in a large bowl. Measure 400ml/14fl oz hand-warm water, then stir in the yogurt, olive oil and vinegar. Mix into the dry ingredients until a sticky dough comes together – it will look like a thick paste at this point. Cover the bowl loosely with some oiled cling film and leave to rise for an hour somewhere warm-ish.

2 Oil your hands well and shape the dough into six round rolls. Lift on to oiled baking sheets. Cover again with oiled cling film and leave for another hour.

3 Heat oven to 240C/220C fan/gas 9. Use your fingers to press a dent in the middle of each roll. Scatter over the roasted peppers, cheese and olives, pressing down into the dents, then finish with the rocket. Drizzle with a little more oil mixed with a good pinch of dried oregano and seasoning. Bake for 20–25 minutes, then put in a large plastic sandwich bag to cool to help soften the crust.

PER ROLL 400 kcals, protein 13g, carbs 63g, fat 12g, sat fat 3g, fibre 3g, sugar 1.6g, salt 2.3g

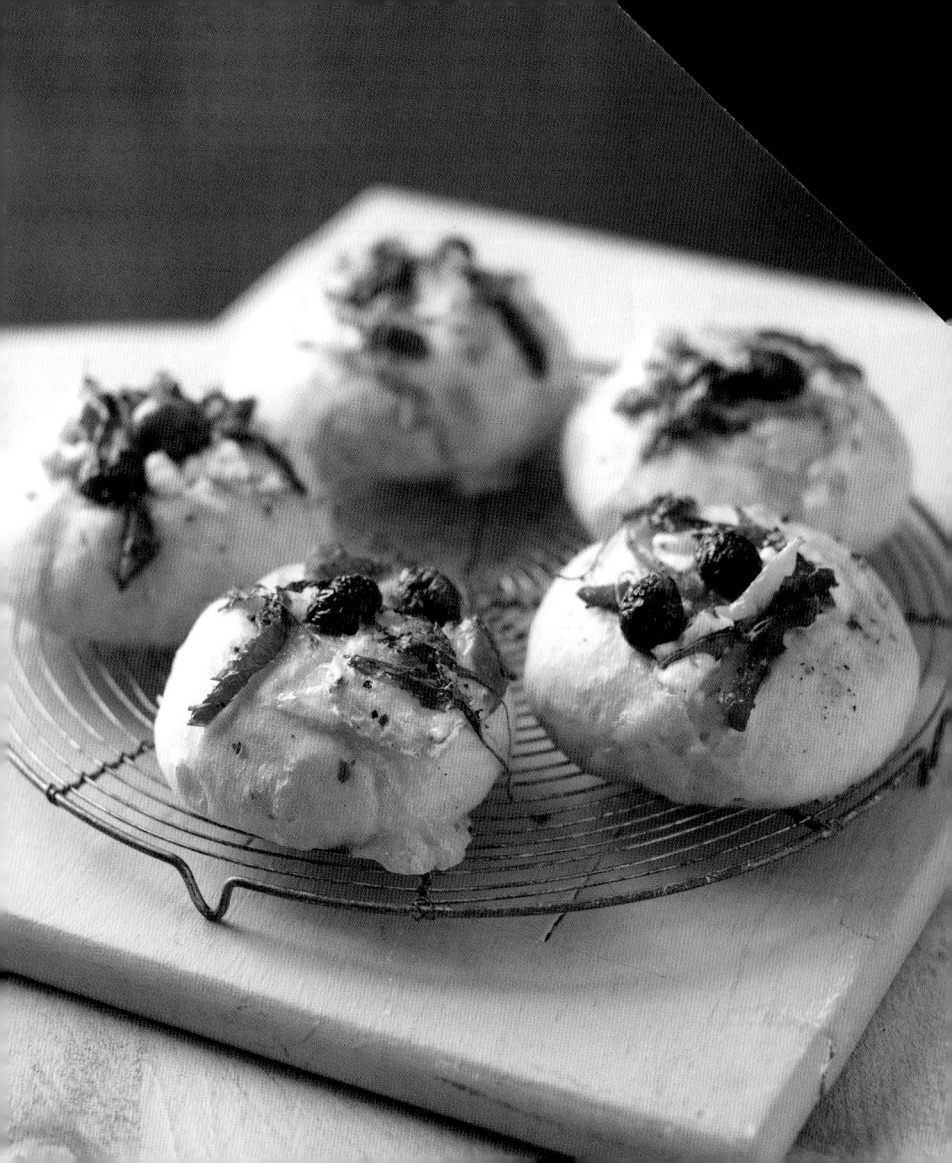

iscuits

n flavours, try sprinkling over a teaspoon of fennel seeds
blespoonfuls of sesame seeds to the mix.

KES 18

flour, plus

½ tsp gluten-free baking powder
50g/2oz cold butter, cut into cubes
1½ tsp flaky sea salt

1 Heat oven to 180C/160C fan/gas 4. Line two baking sheets with baking parchment. Put the flour, xanthan gum, baking powder, butter and ½ teaspoon of the flaky salt in a food processor and whizz for a minute until the butter is completely mixed with the flour. Add 6–8 tablespoons water and pulse until the dough comes together. If it still feels dry, add a teaspoon more water and pulse until you have a soft but not sticky dough.
2 Roll out the dough on a lightly floured surface into a rectangle about 50 × 25cm/20 × 10in and as thin as possible. Brush a little water over the surface of the dough, scatter over 1 teaspoon salt flakes and press in lightly. Prick the dough all over with a fork, then cut into 18 squares. Put on the sheets. Bake for 20 minutes until the biscuits feel dry and sandy but are still pale – they may still feel soft but will harden up when cool. Transfer to a wire rack and leave until cool. Will keep in an airtight container for 2 weeks.

PER BISCUIT 59 kcals, protein 1g, carbs 9g, fat 2g, sat fat 2g, fibre none, sugar none, salt 0.36g

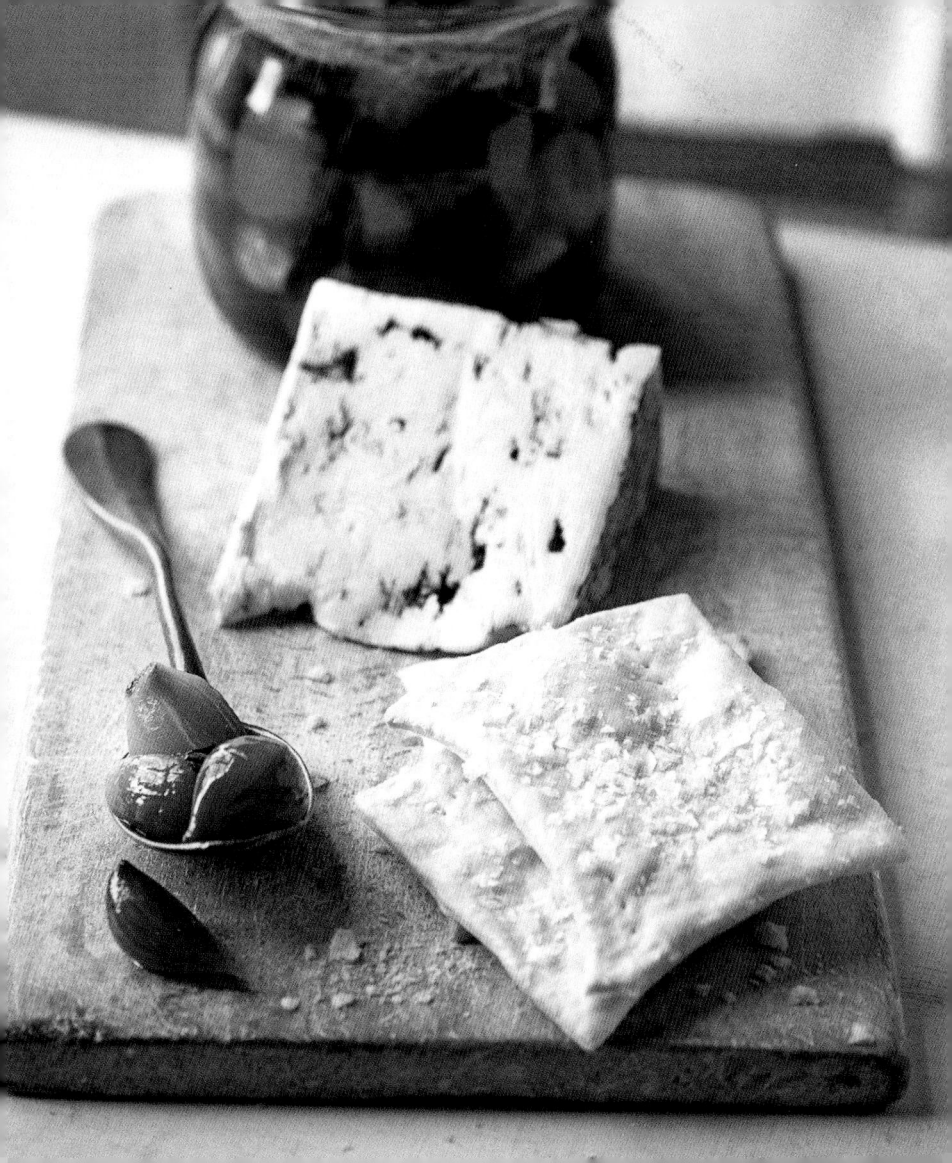

Spinach & potato pies

Half pie, half pasty, these are so good it's worth organising a picnic just as an excuse to bake up a batch! Enjoy warm, or cold.

TAKES 1 HOUR 20 MINUTES
- **MAKES 8**

200g/7oz spinach leaves
1 small baking potato, peeled, cut into
    small chunks and boiled until tender
150ml pot single cream
1 egg, beaten
100g/4oz Cheddar, grated
grated fresh nutmeg

FOR THE PASTRY

140g/5oz buckwheat flour
140g/5oz gluten-free plain flour, plus
    extra for dusting
2 tbsp bran
1 tsp xanthan gum
140g/5oz cold butter, diced
2 eggs, beaten separately

1 First make the pastry. Rub the flours, bran and xanthan gum together with the butter to the texture of breadcrumbs. Mix one egg with 1 tablespoon water, then work in until a pastry comes together. Knead the pastry on a work surface until soft. Chill for 1 hour.

2 Tip the spinach into a colander, pour over boiling water to wilt; squeeze out the liquid. Mix the spinach with the potatoes, cream, egg and two-thirds of the cheese. Season with salt, pepper and nutmeg.

3 Heat oven to 200C/180C fan/gas 6. Roll the pastry out on a floured surface to the thickness of a £1 coin. Cut out eight 13cm/5in squares. Spoon the mix into the centre of each square, then brush the edges with the second beaten egg. Bring all four corners together over the filling, pinching the edges together to make a sealed purse. Sit on baking sheets.

4 Brush each pie with the remaining egg, then top with remaining grated cheese. Bake for 30 minutes until golden.

PER PIE 421 kcals, protein 11g, carbs 31g, fat 31g, sat fat 11g, fibre 3g, sugar 2g, salt 0.57g

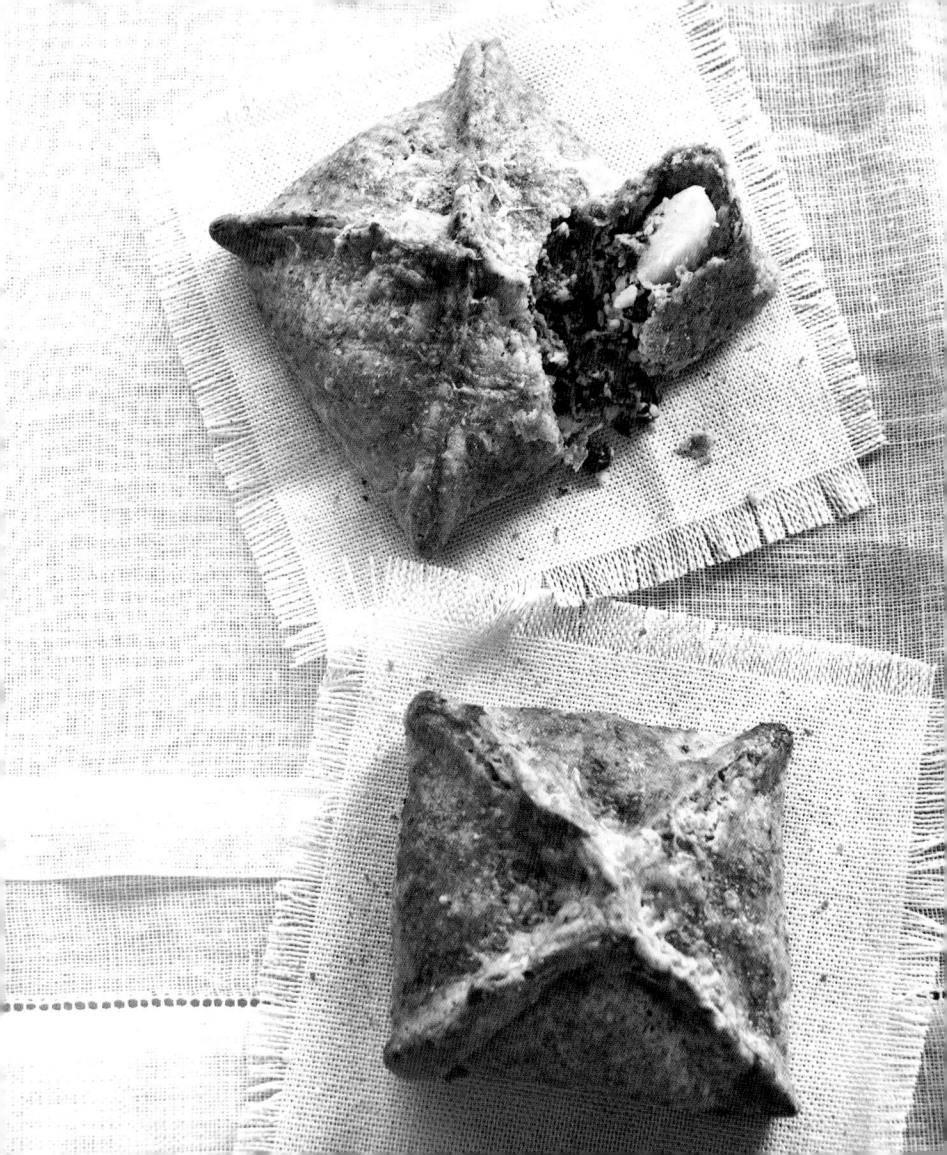

Potato pancakes

Eggs, bacon, smoked salmon or baked beans, these savoury pancakes will go with just about anything, so gather up the family for Sunday brunch.

TAKES 45 MINUTES ● MAKES 12–15

75g/2½oz gluten-free plain flour
1 tsp gluten-free baking powder
250g/9oz cold mashed potato
2 eggs
125ml/4fl oz milk
1 rounded tbsp finely snipped chives
sunflower oil
few knobs of butter
your favourite accompaniments,
    to serve

1 Sieve the flour and baking powder on to the mash. Whisk the eggs and milk together, and add to the potato mix with the chives. Whisk the batter until smooth.
3 Heat a large non-stick frying pan over a medium heat. Add ½ teaspoon sunflower oil and a dot of butter. When the fat is hot, start to cook the pancakes. Add 1 tablespoon of batter for each pancake and cook about four at a time. Cook for about 1 minute until the underside is golden brown and small bubbles appear.
4 Flip the pancakes and cook until golden. Remove from the pan and keep warm while you cook the remaining pancakes in the same way, adding a tiny bit of oil and butter to the pan as and when needed. Serve the pancakes in stacks with scrambled egg and streaky bacon, smoked salmon and hollandaise, or baked beans and gluten-free sausages.

PER SERVING 75 kcals, protein 3g, carbs 9g, fat 3g, sat fat 1g, fibre none, sugar 0.7g, salt 0.20g

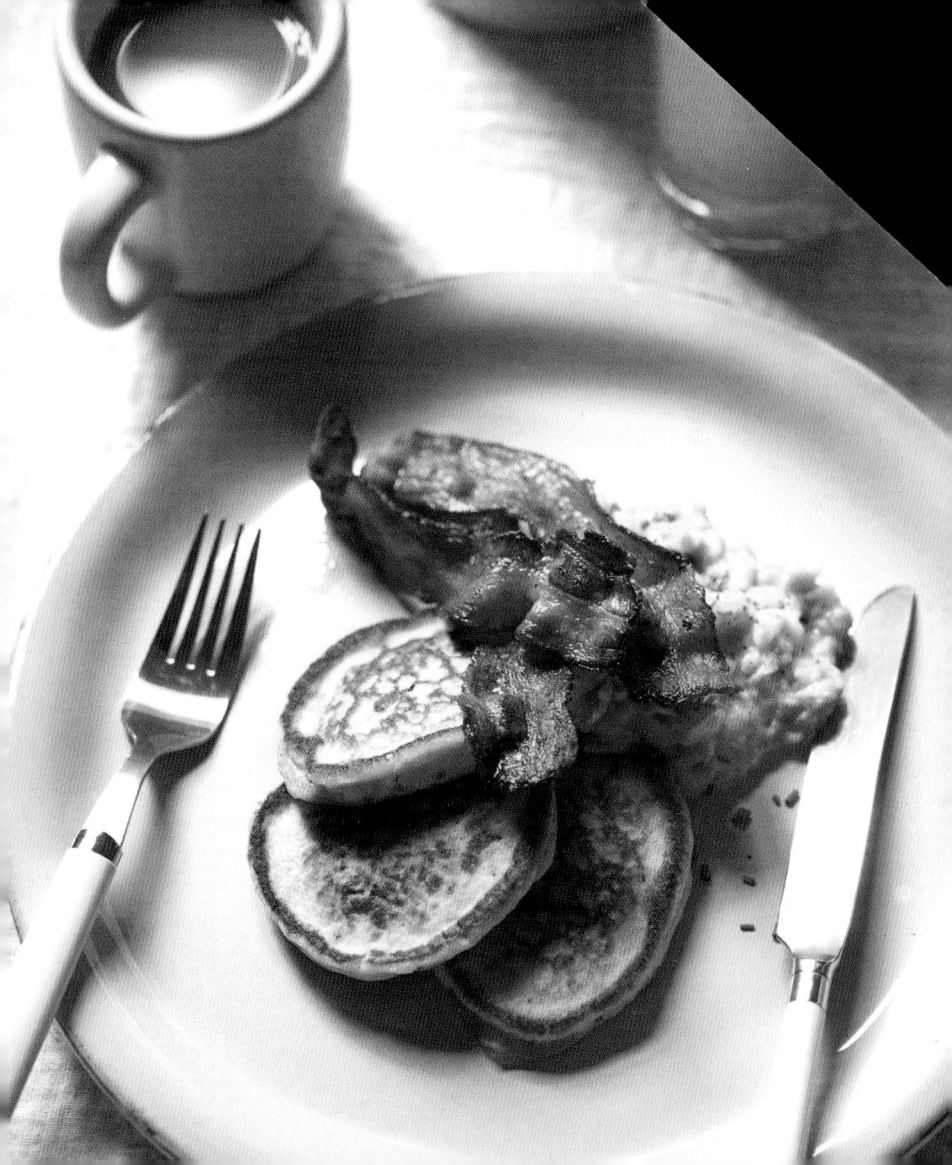

n quiche

ese pizza, well here's a three-cheese tart – a delicious way to cheeseboard.

UTES

FOR THE PASTRY

300g/10oz gluten-free flour, plus extra
   for rolling
1 tsp xanthan gum
140g/5oz cold butter, diced
1 egg, beaten

FOR THE FILLING

2 onions, sliced into rings
1 tbsp oil
2 large eggs
284ml pot double cream
250g/9oz cheese (we used ⅓ each
   Stilton, Brie and Cheddar)

1 Make the pastry according to the method on p82.

2 Heat oven to 200C/180C fan/gas 6. Roll the pastry out on a floured surface until large enough to line a 23cm loose-bottomed tart tin. Line the tin with the pastry, leaving any excess pastry overhanging. Line with greaseproof paper, then fill with baking beans. Bake on a baking sheet for 15 minutes. Take out the paper and beans, then bake for 10 minutes more until pale golden and cooked.

3 While the pastry cooks, gently soften the onions in the oil until golden. Beat the eggs and cream together, then season to taste. Crumble up the hard cheeses and chop or pull the creamy cheese into small pieces. Scatter the cheese into the pastry case, add the onions, then pour in the egg mix. Turn the oven down to 160C/140C fan/gas 3 and bake for 40 minutes until set and lightly golden.

PER SERVING 603 kcals, protein 13g, carbs 30g, fat 49g, sat fat 26g, fibre 2g, sugar 5g, salt 1.18g

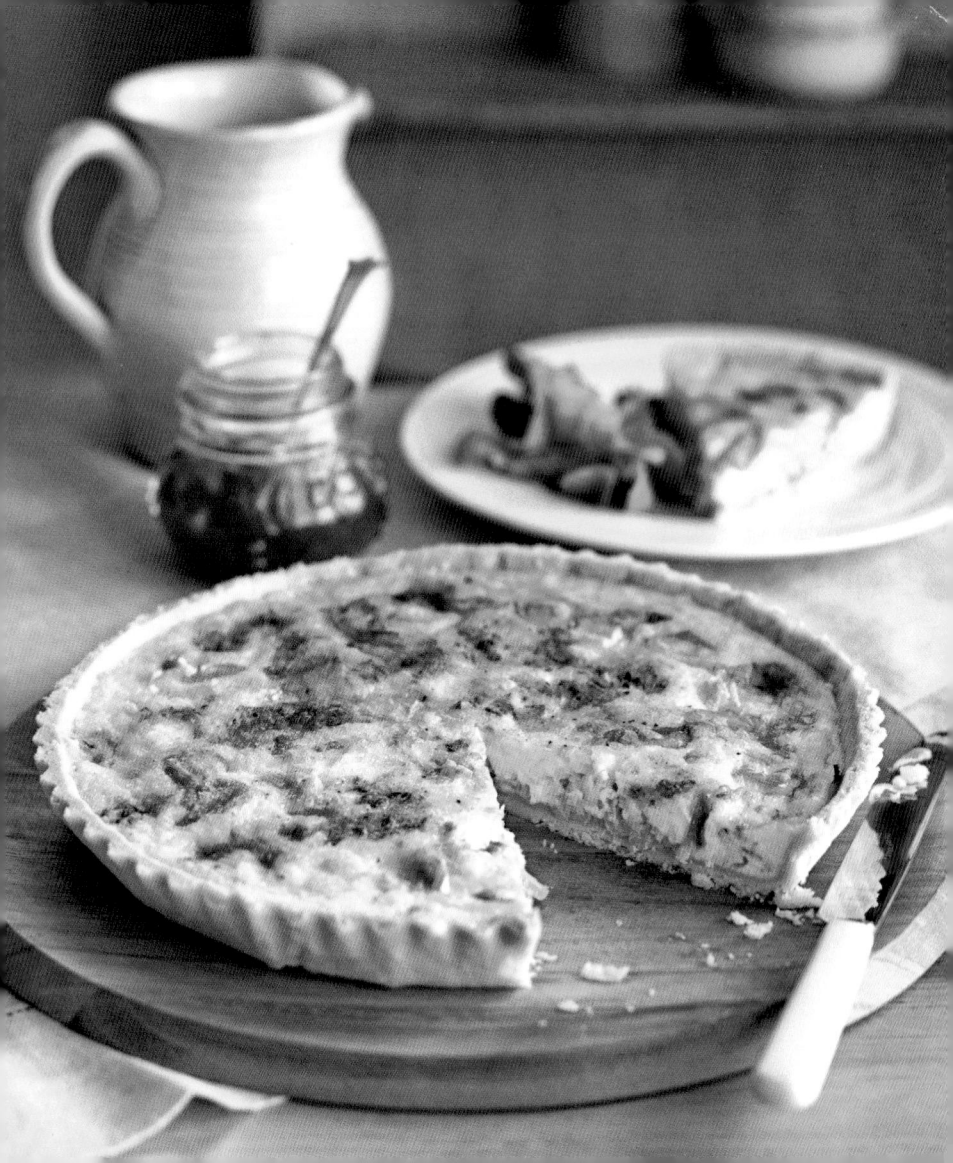

Cornish pasties

The black pepper is essential in this recipe, giving the pasties their spicy kick.

TAKES 1 HOUR 20 MINUTES, PLUS CHILLING • MAKES 4

FOR THE PASTRY

120g/4½oz cold butter, diced
120g/4½oz cold lard, diced
500g/1lb 2oz gluten-free plain flour, plus extra for rolling
2 tsp xanthan gum
1 egg, beaten, to seal and glaze

FOR THE FILLING

350g/12oz beef skirt or chuck steak, finely chopped
1 large onion, finely chopped
2 medium potatoes, peeled and thinly sliced
175g/6oz swede, peeled and finely diced
1 tbsp freshly ground black pepper

1 Rub the butter and lard into the flour and xanthan gum with a pinch of salt using your fingertips or a food processor, then blend in 6 tablespoons cold water to make a firm dough. Briefly knead, cut equally into four, then chill for 20 minutes.

2 Heat oven to 220C/200C fan/gas 7. Mix together the filling ingredients with 1 teaspoon salt. Roll out each piece of dough on a lightly floured surface until large enough to make a round about 23cm/9in wide – use a plate to trim it to shape. Firmly pack a quarter of the filling along the centre of each round, leaving a margin at each end. Brush the pastry all the way round the edge with beaten egg, carefully draw up both sides so that they meet at the top, then pinch them together to seal. Lift on to a non-stick baking sheet and brush with the remaining egg to glaze.

3 Bake for 10 minutes, then lower oven to 180C/160C fan/gas 4 and cook for 45 minutes more until golden. Great served warm.

PER PASTY 1,174 kcals, protein 34g, carbs 114g, fat 68g, sat fat 35g, fibre 6g, sugar 7g, salt 1.96g

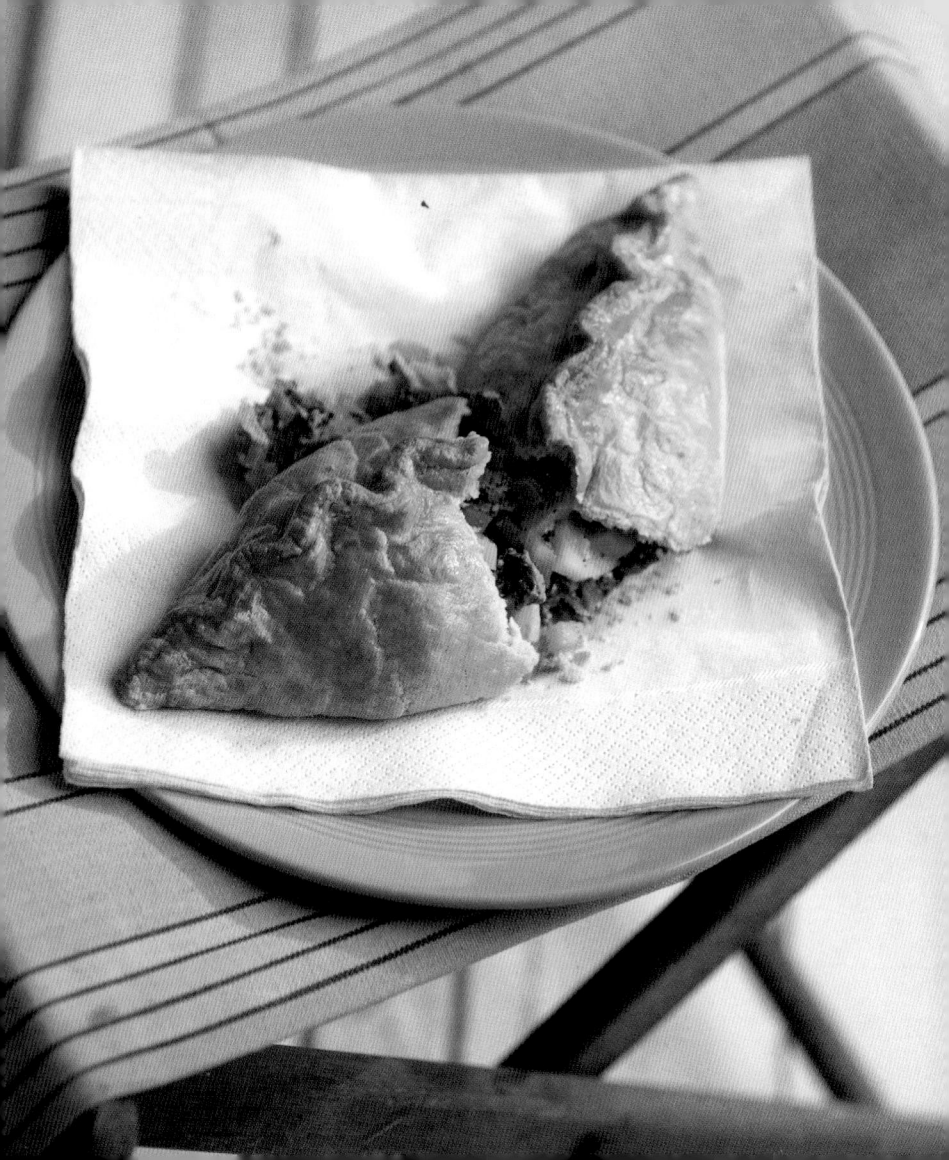

Pepper pissaladière

You can use any colour of peppers for this, but red, yellow or orange will give this dish a much brighter appearance than green.

TAKES 1¾ HOURS • **SERVES 4**

2 Spanish onions, finely sliced

3 fat garlic cloves, finely sliced

4 peppers, deseeded and sliced

4 tbsp olive oil, plus a little more for drizzling (optional)

2 handfuls pitted green or black olives, quartered

2 tbsp capers, rinsed and drained

6 anchovies, each cut into 4 long strips (optional)

FOR THE DOUGH

450g/1lb gluten-free plain flour, plus extra for rolling

2 tsp xanthan gum

2 tsp caster sugar

1 × 7g sachet fast-action dried yeast

2 eggs, beaten

6 tbsp olive oil, plus extra for greasing

1 Heat oven to 200C/180C fan/gas 6. Tip the onions, garlic, peppers and olive oil into a roasting tin and cook for 40–45 minutes, stirring occasionally, until the onions and peppers are soft and tinged brown. Stir in the olives and capers, and season well.

2 Meanwhile, for the dough, mix the flour, gum, sugar, yeast and 1 teaspoon salt in a bowl. Make a well in the centre and add the eggs, oil and 250ml/9fl oz hand-warm water, and stir with a wooden spoon to a sticky dough. Knead for 5 minutes on a floured surface then sit in an oiled bowl, cover with a clean tea towel and leave in a warm-ish place to rise for 30 minutes.

3 Roll and press the dough out to fit a baking sheet, about 40 × 30cm. Spoon over the topping mix. Press gently into the dough and scatter over the anchovies, if using.

4 Bake for 25–30 minutes or until the dough has risen and cooked through. Drizzle with olive oil to serve, if you like.

PER SERVING 306 kcals, protein 7g, carbs 38g, fat 15g, sat fat 2g, fibre 6g, sugar 15g, salt 2.3g

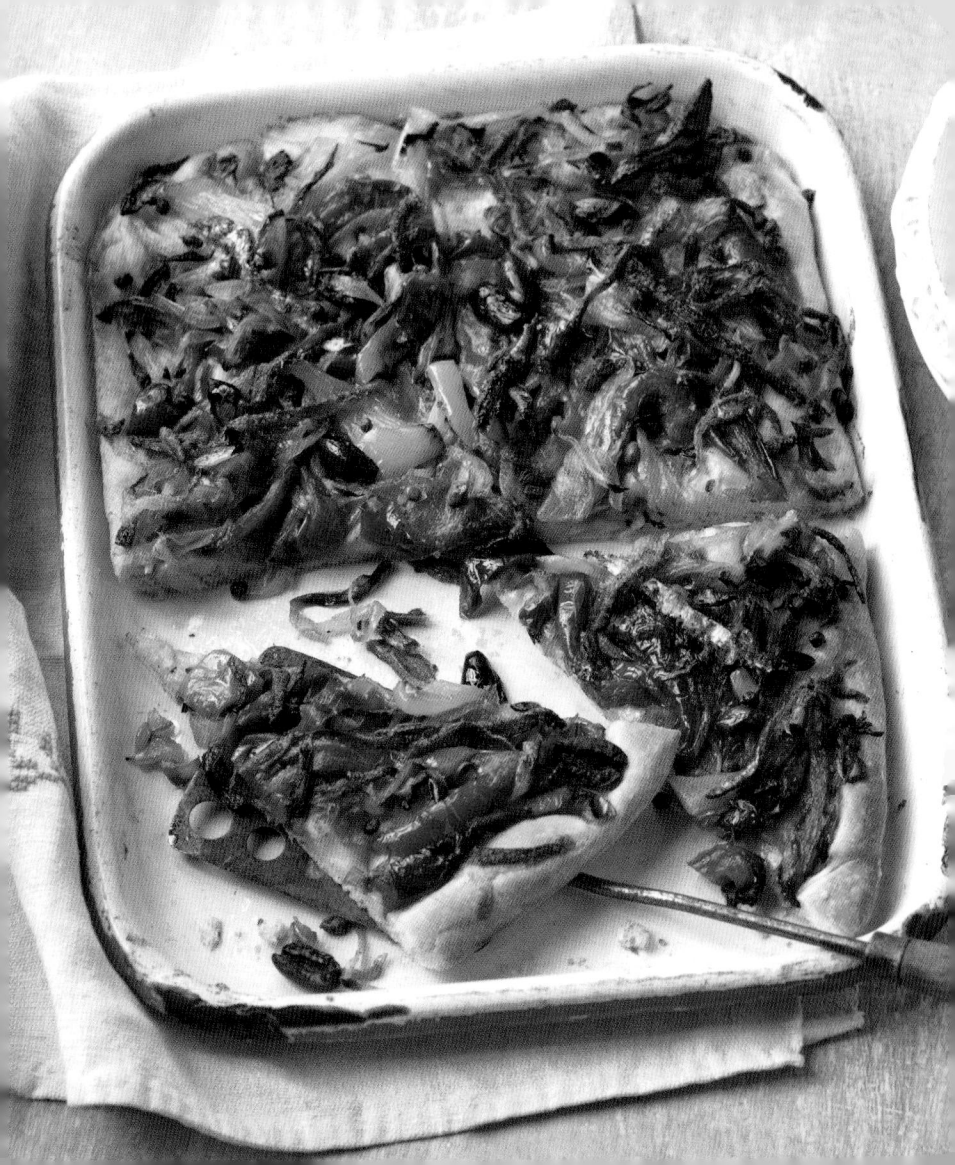

Index

Also available from BBC Books and *Good Food*

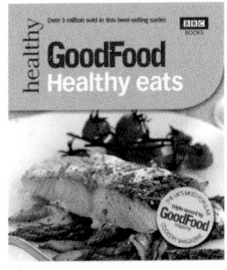
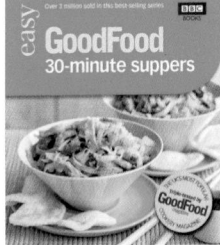
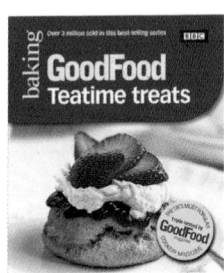
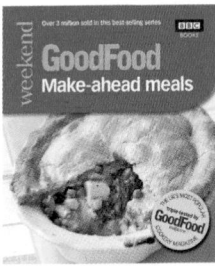
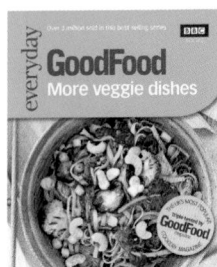
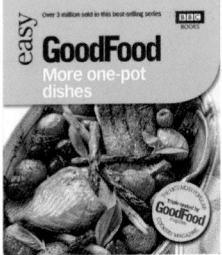

Subscribe for £10.50! *

Good Food is now available on iPad as a digital-only subscription.

- Subscribe for 6 months and pay just £1.75 per issue, saving you £7.44 on a 6-issue subscription**.

- Each issue is packed with brand-new recipes, including everyday and seasonal meals. Plus get access to the great interactive features of the app – save and email shopping lists, and watch tutorial videos.

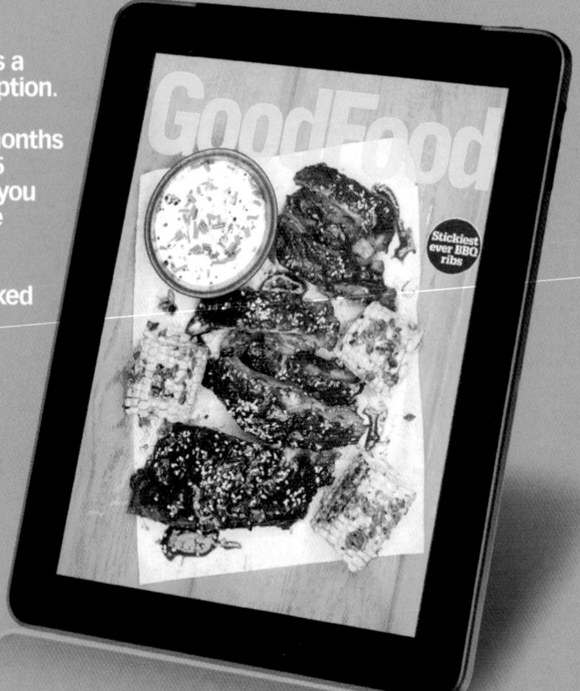

 To get your subscription, and for full terms and conditions, visit *buysubscriptions.com* and click on 'Digital Titles'.